Dr. Kushner's Personality Type Diet

Robert F. Kushner, M.D.,
and Nancy Kushner, M.S.N., R.N.

Recipes by Eileen Vincent, M.S., R.D., L.D.

St. Martin's Griffin ᛗ
New York

www.stmartins.com

BOOK DESIGN BY CAROL MALCOLM RUSSO/SIGNET M DESIGN, INC.

Library of Congress Cataloging-in-Publication Data

Kushner, Robert F., 1953–
   Dr. Kushner's personality type diet / Robert F. Kushner and Nancy Kushner.—1st ed.
      p. cm.
   Includes bibliographical references (page 288) and index (page 291).
   ISBN 0-312-28809-3 (hc)
   ISBN 0-312-32582-7 (pbk)
   1. Weight loss. 2. Food habits. 3. Personality. I. Title: Doctor Kushner's personality type diet. II. Title: Personality type diet. III. Kushner, Nancy. IV. Title.

RM222.2 .K868 2003
613.7'—dc21

2002033281

First St. Martin's Griffin Edition: January 2004

10 9 8 7 6 5 4 3 2 1

"Thanks to *Dr. Kushner's Personality Type Diet*, staying slim just got easier. If you're looking for a weight loss program that promises to boost your motivation and metabolism, this book is for you."

—Miriam E. Nelson, Ph.D.
Bestselling author of *Strong Women Stay Slim* and *Strong Women Stay Young*

"Dr. Kushner brings fresh emphasis to the spectrum of colorful foods that dieters should put on their plates and into their stomachs to achieve healthy weight loss. And his lifestyle pattern approach will benefit many dieters by pointing the way toward achieving and maintaining a healthy body weight."

—David Heber, M.D., Ph.D, professor of medicine, UCLA, director
of the UCLA Center for Human Nutrition, and author of *What Color Is Your Diet?*

"If you can't see Dr. Kushner yourself, buy this book! He has made it possible to recognize and overcome all major pitfalls that dieters encounter."

—Louis Aronne, M.D., clinical associate professor of medicine,
Joan and Sanford I. Weill Medical College of Cornell University

"This book is supersized with great ideas for scaling down. The recipes and menu suggestions are sound and tasty . . . and the three-week-starter plan is sure to jump-start even those who feel they can't lose weight. BRAVO."

—Michael F. Roizen, M.D.
Bestselling author of *RealAge* and *The RealAge Diet*

"Read this book. You'll discover your eating and exercise types, as well as sound, surefooted ways to change them. Dr. Kushner, one of our nation's leading experts in weight control, provides recipes for the mind, body, and soul."

—Thomas A. Wadden, Ph.D., director of the Weight and Eating Disorders Program,
University of Pennsylvania School of Medicine

"*Dr. Kushner's Personality Type Diet* is a welcome book for people trying to lose weight. Rather than a 'one size fits all' approach, Dr. Kushner shows you how to find the right weight loss strategy for you. This book should help many people be successful in long-term weight loss maintenance."

—James O. Hill, Ph.D., director of the Center for Human Nutrition,
University of Colorado Health Science Center

"This book will strike a chord with anyone who knows how challenging it can be to manage weight. Dr. Kushner shows us how our own personalities along with a permissive environment can promote weight gain. More important, he provides practical and scientifically sound advice to help people do something about it."

—Donald D. Hensrud, M.D., M.Ph., associate professor of preventive medicine and nutrition, Mayo Medical School, and editor in chief of *Mayo Clinic on Healthy Weight*

*To our parents and children, who enrich our lives
and inspire us to enrich the lives of others*

Note to the Reader

The names and attributes of the patients mentioned in this book have been changed to protect their anonymity. In some cases, patient descriptions are a composite of patients with similar stories. This book is a source of information and is not intended as a substitute for medical care. Consult with a qualified medical professional before embarking on this or any new weight loss program.

Dr. Kushner would like to hear from you. You may E-mail your comments, feedback, and weight loss experience to doctorkushner@aol.com. Visit his Web site at www.DoctorKushner.com

Contents

Acknowledgments

R obert Kushner thanks his patients for sharing their life stories, thoughtful words of wisdom, and personal insights. They can take pride in knowing that the ideas of this book were created from their individual struggles and successes with weight loss and will, in turn, help everyone who reads this book.

The staff at the Wellness Institute at Northwestern Memorial Hospital in Chicago has provided invaluable advice and assistance. In particular, we want to acknowledge registered dietitian Dawn Jackson for her creative and motivating diet and nutrition ideas, psychologist Johanna Mytko for her expert assistance with the coping strategies and developing and analyzing the Diet Personality Quiz, psychologist Cindy Levin for her perceptiveness and attentiveness to the coping strategies, and exercise physiologist Peggy Mitchell for her important suggestions regarding the exercise strategies. Patients in the Wellness Institute benefited from the patterns approach to weight management through instruction by our highly talented and professional staff members, who include registered dietitians Amy Baltes, Barbara Eichorst, Laurie Maimonis, and Judy Quinn; physicians Edith Ramsdell and Hazel Manzano; exercise specialist Kristen Peterson, and health educator Javon Pelt. We are deeply appreciative of their enthusiasm for and belief in this new treatment approach and all of their hard work in implementing it into the Wellness Institute.

We also want to thank Eileen Vincent, a registered dietitian and research nutritionist at the Feinberg School of Medicine, Northwestern University, for developing her super foods concept to create the thirty delicious recipes—complete with nutrition analyses, menu plans, and companion nutrient and health benefits tables. Eileen taught us a lot about the art and science of cooking with super foods, not only to lose weight but also to boost health. Her attention to detail ensured that each recipe was tested, retested, and then perfected until it met with the approval of her taste testers (thanks especially to John). As this recipe project seemed to take on a life of its own, Eileen handled it with great ease and a professional spirit. We thank her for that.

A good editor and agent make their authors look better. We were lucky to have both. A big thank you to our editor, Heather Jackson Silverman, who believed in our project from the start and gave us sound advice all along the way. Her kind, considerate manner and editorial wisdom were deeply appreciated. We are indebted to our agent, Caroline Carney of Book Deals, who, like a personal stylist, trimmed, cut, and sharpened our manuscript until it was ready to take on the road. A course that can be tedious for some authors instead became a process of discovery and growth with Caroline's support, encouragement, and expertise. In addition, we would like to thank the following people, who shared their professional insights with us: Maija Balagot, Susan Berger Kabaker, Gary Kash, and Jim Kepler.

We would also like to thank our parents for their continual love and support and our extended family of siblings, nieces, and nephews, who spent many holiday celebrations trying to think of a title. Thank you to our friends, and especially the members of our fun club, who gave us a welcome relief from spending long hours in front of the computer by helping us stay active. Finally, we thank our children, Sarah and Steve, for their patience and good humor during endless hours of taste testing and discussion of fiber food facts at the dinner table.

Introduction

■ ■ ■ ■ ■

This is not your typical diet book and I am not your typical physician. The program in this book is a medically sound one that has already changed the lives of my patients. It works because, having listened to thousands of patients talk about the struggles they faced as dieters, I developed a program based on their experiences, which provides real answers and solutions to life's challenges. My twenty-year journey of listening, learning, and discovering has culminated in the Personality Type Diet.

I first became interested in nutrition and weight control as a fourth-year medical student because I was truly moved by the frustration that dieters felt as they tried one diet after another without success. I also was fascinated with the intricacies of metabolism and appetite control that underlie many of the medical treatments available today. After finishing a residency in internal medicine, I completed a two-year postgraduate fellowship in nutrition and a master's degree in nutrition. This was as rare a career path for physicians back then as it is today. In 1984, I began to treat patients burdened by overweight and obesity by establishing the first multidisciplinary weight management program at the University of Chicago. In 1998, I moved the program to Northwestern University and assumed the position of medical director of the Wellness Institute at Northwestern Memorial Hospital in Chicago. Here I embraced the importance of the mind-body connection to healthy weight loss, which complements my more traditional and science-based medical training. I also made some new discoveries that forever changed my approach to weight management and spearheaded this book.

As a medical student, I was always trained to listen to my patients' symptoms and then direct my treatment toward improving those symptoms. For example, a patient with asthma who complains of nighttime wheezing requires a different treatment plan from someone with exercise-induced asthma. Yet the traditional approach to helping patients lose weight didn't vary with "symptoms" as much as in other diseases. As I paid more attention to my patients' symptoms of being overweight, I noticed definite patterns. One patient was a night eater, another used food to deal with stress, and yet another liked to exercise but couldn't fit it into her busy schedule. These lifestyle patterns (or "symptom patterns" as I identify them to other physicians) have helped to form the foundation for this revolutionary personality approach to weight control.

In brief, this approach helps you to identify your diet personality—which eating, exercise, and coping lifestyle patterns have been preventing you from losing weight for good. Using simple quizzes and checklists, you learn to zero in on the lifestyle patterns that continually trip you up, and you learn the step-by-step weight-busting strategies to overcome them. Like peeling the layers of an onion, you will discover how to shape one pattern, enjoy the benefits, and then move on to the next. I simplify and personalize a weight management program that can be woven painlessly into each of your busy lives.

I often reflect on how much my patients have taught me about weight control—specifically what works for them and what doesn't. Their responses to my treatment approach through the years have helped make my program what it is today. I'd like to share with you some patient comments that support seven weight management prescriptions that are central to my program.

Rx 1: Stop Blaming Yourself

Previously I had always blamed myself for being overweight—thinking there was something wrong with me. But after being in your program, now I really understand why my weight has been out of control; it's the environment we live in.

Over the years, as I noticed the similarities in my patients' struggles with weight loss and regain, I realized there were strong environmental forces pressuring patients to eat more and exercise less. I even coined a term that explains it: scaling up syndrome. In Chapter 1, you learn why you have struggled with losing weight and keeping it off. As you better understand the real culprit in the battle of the bulge, your energies can be directed away from self-blame and toward weight loss and improved health. And for those interested in jump-starting their weight loss, I provide a special three-week plan.

Rx 2: Know Your Lifestyle

Many doctors have suggested that I needed to change my lifestyle, handed me a written, low-calorie diet to follow, then sent me on my way. But you actually taught me how to change my lifestyle, and you did it in such a gradual way that I didn't notice it happening and it really wasn't hard.

My patients taught me early on that the solution to controlling weight once and for all doesn't lie in following a preprinted diet plan or unsound, unscientific, and silly "food rules" but rather with a better understanding of themselves and their particular lifestyle. That's why in Chapter 2, I help you to identify the eating, exercise, and coping patterns that have fed your weight gain. These three aspects of your diet personality form the foundation for my personalized treatment plans that follow. Once you understand the patterns that have caused weight gain, you can take back control to reshape them, one pattern at a time.

Rx 3: Make Small Changes

When I started your program, weight loss seemed to be such a huge, insurmountable hurdle. I didn't know what to do first, but you were able to break it up into manageable pieces for me.

Since my patients' lives are so busy, I knew that big lifestyle changes would never work for them over the long run. Instead it was the small, easy-to-follow changes that added up to make the biggest differences in their weight and health. In Chapters 3, 4, and 5, you learn the simple steps (tailored to your particular eating, exercise, and coping patterns) that will help you achieve the long-term success you've been seeking.

Rx 4: Self-Monitor to Stay on Track

With all other weight loss programs, I'd lose the weight and then gain it right back. But your self-monitoring tools and strategies enabled me to catch a temporary lapse in behaviors and prevent it from turning into total collapse.

Lapses in behavior are an expected part of any weight loss program. The key is to identify them early so you can troubleshoot and then take the corrective actions that put you back in control. In Chapter 6, you learn the three-step process for weight maintenance along with ways your family and friends can support your long-term successes.

Rx 5: Identify Recipes for Success

I always thought that cooking healthy was time-consuming and difficult to master. But after trying the right recipes, I was happily proved wrong.

Learning how to cook healthful, good-tasting foods is a valuable skill—especially if you want to reach and maintain your weight loss goal. But you need the right recipes. Developed by a registered dietitian, who is also a healthy cooking expert, the recipes and menu plans in Chapter 7 are sure to be big hits at your table.

Rx 6: Be Resourceful

When it comes to my general health care needs, I usually make good choices, but when it comes to weight loss, I am frequently confused. Whether I needed psychological counseling, dietary guidance, or medical interventions, you always steered me right.

Part of being successful on a healthy weight loss program is being able to identify if and when you need additional help. Since the process of losing weight may require you to have more extensive dietary counseling (for example, if you have diabetes or food intolerances), or can expose sensitive issues (depression or binge eating disorder) that are helped by psychological counseling or can be supported by physician monitoring and intervention, you need to know your options. In Chapter 8, you learn the different resources available if you ever need them.

The Bottom Line

The bottom line to my beliefs about weight control and this book is that weight management is about so much more than just carbs and protein. It's your lifestyle that holds the key to conquering your weight loss struggles. So my book's mission is threefold.

- First, to help you understand how scaling up syndrome has played out in your life.
- Second, to help you identify your particular diet personality—that is, the unconscious eating, exercise, and coping patterns you've developed in response to this syndrome.
- Third, to guide you step by step to reshape your lifestyle patterns toward healthy, lasting weight loss.

As I tell my patients, we're in this together—and for the long run.

How to Use This Book

Though your typical diet book approach may be to skip the beginning chapters and fast-forward to the later chapters, I don't recommend this because you'll be missing out on the process of awareness and self-discovery that forms the foundation of this program. And I also highly recommend that you try the three-week starter plan that allows you to begin the process of behavior change while also jump-starting your mind and body toward weight loss and improved health. Once you complete (and then tally) your diet personality quiz in Chapter 2, you'll have a couple of options. You can either zero in on the specific sections in Chapters 3–5 that pertain to your identified patterns, or you can read through the chapters in their entirety, learning about all the patterns (before you go back to focus on your own). By doing the latter, you'll learn all the weight loss strategies that have helped my patients over the years. You'll also be more knowledgeable about how scaling up syndrome can affect members of your family, colleagues at work, and friends—or even you, maybe at a later date. Since your diet personality can change alongside your life challenges, this book is meant to be a living document for successful weight loss that you can turn to for help again and again.

■   ■   ■   ■   ■

Dr. Kushner's
Personality
Type
Diet

Chapter 1

Scaling Up Syndrome

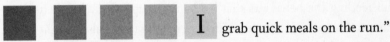I grab quick meals on the run."

"I eat out a lot."

"I don't have time to cook like I used to."

"I know I need to work out, but I'm too tired."

"I'm really stressed out."

"I can't lose weight."

If these patient statements sound familiar, you may also have symptoms of scaling up syndrome.

Throughout my years of practice, I have observed many highly successful patients who have climbed corporate ladders, managed large households and budgets, raised productive children, and volunteered their time to better society—and yet they still were not successful at taking care of their health and losing weight. Their passions were being directed toward their jobs, their families, and their financial futures, and they had lost touch with their personal needs.

After listening to thousands of these dieters' stories, I began to detect a clear pattern to their weight management struggles. Soon I realized this pattern was really a syndrome that can and must be treated before someone can lose weight for good. I coined a term that explains it: scaling up syndrome. Certain benefits of our society in excess—the open opportunity to be self-made; the wide availability of cheap, convenient food; the easy access to labor-saving technology—secretly sabotage our innate desire to look and feel good. For instance, the chance to achieve the American dream becomes a driving, stressful pressure to work harder and longer, while the omnipresence of rich restaurant, snack, and fast food in plentiful portions becomes a welcome invitation to take a break and "treat yourself." Further, in response to these societal pressures, many people have developed unconscious eating, exercise, and coping patterns that also lead to their accumulation of excess pounds, which I call "false weight."

Why do I call the 10, 20, 30, or 50 + pounds that someone unconsciously gains as a consequence of scaling up syndrome false weight? If you took that same person and changed only her environment—perhaps you moved her to Paris for a few years where walking is a major mode of transportation and small portions of food are common—this particular weight would scale down (or decrease) and might even melt completely away. Absent the societal stimuli feeding the behaviors that led to the weight gain, her behaviors would shift and her weight would reduce. In other words, false weight is not weight resulting from genetics or metabolism or natural appetite or frame size or even low willpower: It is weight resulting from an unconscious adaptation to the multifaceted pressures of modern society.

For one patient it was the freshman 10, the stressful job 6, the honeymoon 4, and the baby 8—totaling a gain of 28 pounds of false weight. For another, it was the long commute 8 and the divorce 15—totaling a gain of 23 pounds of false weight. And for still another it was a death in the family 18, a desk job 10, and a layoff 6—totaling a gain of 34 pounds of false weight. You may wonder if all of these patients shared some genetic predisposition to becoming overweight as they matured through their adult lives. In fact, none of them had a genetic disorder, but they did all suffer from the same syndrome that affects the majority of overweight Americans today: scaling up syndrome. This syndrome is insidious, as it strikes hardworking men and women who are busy trying to get ahead in each area of their life. But with each passing year and each new responsibility, their health has been put on the back burner. Maybe they've tried a crash diet here or there, but their day-to-day life stresses always win over this short-lived approach. As quickly as they start a diet, they stop it and then forget about their health—until the next enticing crash diet comes along. And as this ineffective cycle repeats itself, their false weight gain grows paradoxically along with their life accomplishments.

Your Authentic Shape vs. False Weight

Though many patients come to me when they're at their wit's end regarding their weight, it doesn't take me long (usually within the first visit) to help them achieve a breakthrough. After a medical checkup and inventory of their diet history, I ask patients to look at how their life events have affected their weight gain. I'm going to ask you to do the same thing so you can see how scaling up syndrome has played out in your life. This awareness is a crucial first step in your journey toward shedding the weight you've accumulated over the years and toward recovering your authentic shape—which is the weight range and fitness level at which you feel the healthiest, most energetic, and most attractive.

Think about yourself and how your weight has climbed to where it's at today. Let the following table help you to recall the pounds you gained (or lost) that may relate to specific life events. Begin this exercise by first writing down your approximate weight at age 18 and your current weight.

Approximate weight at age 18: _160_ Current weight: _196_

Now in the table below, fill in the approximate number of pounds gained or lost along with the net weight change during each decade of life. If in your thirties, for example, you gained 35 pounds but lost 10, then your net weight gain for that time period becomes +25 pounds. Think about the life events that occurred during each time span that may relate to your weight changes and write them in as well. These life events may include (but not be limited to):

- breaking up with a boyfriend or girlfriend
- quitting smoking, drinking, or drug use
- moving to a new location like a college dorm or a new community
- getting married or divorced
- starting a new job, changing jobs, getting fired, or retiring from your job
- having children
- caring for your family
- becoming an empty nester
- enduring death or illness in the family
- suffering from an illness

- having money problems
- some other traumatic or even successful life event that you relate to gaining or losing weight

Number of Pounds of Weight Gained (or Lost) and Life Events

Age	Life Events	Weight Changes
18–20s		___ lbs. gained ___ lbs. lost ___ net wt. change
30s	*having children, family, job*	*15* lbs. gained ___ lbs. lost *15* net wt. change
40s	*chair position*	*10* lbs. gained ___ lbs. lost *10* net wt. change
50s	*gaining weight*	*11* lbs. gained ___ lbs. lost *11* net wt. change
60s+		___ lbs. gained ___ lbs. lost ___ net wt. change

Now, record the total weight gained over the years: *36*

If you feel that your weight gain is overwhelming, you may benefit from hearing words of encouragement I typically give patients at this point in the program. Since it probably has taken years or decades for your weight to climb up the ladder to where it is today, now is the time to work your way back down the ladder. As you learn the strategies that have worked for my patients, you will understand how strategy by strategy they've been able to build healthy weight loss into their lives. If they can do it, you can too.

> ⇜ *Nibble on This* ⇝
> Resolve that your present weight is the heaviest you will ever weigh.

Many patients have also found it helpful actually to graph the relationship between their life events and their weight, especially since people gain weight in different ways. Some gain in a progressive upward (or ratcheting) fashion, others gain in an up-and-down cyclic or yo-yo fashion, and still others, after a long period of controlled weight, see their weight climb steadily after one inciting event (see the three graph examples below). The more insight you develop regarding your particular weight gain patterns, the better positioned you will be to take back control and reverse them.

Progressive (or Ratcheting) Weight Gain

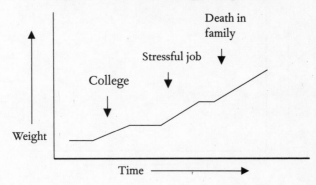

Weight Cycling or Yo-Yo Weight Gain

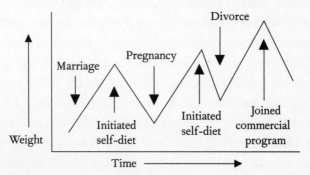

Inciting Event Weight Gain

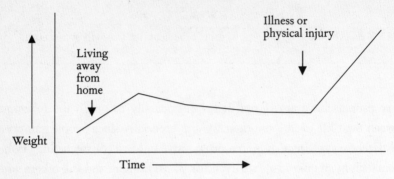

I want you to now graph your own weight gain. Be sure to fill in the life events that you relate to your weight. Take note of your pattern so you can better understand your weight gain, that is, how you got to where you are today.

Your Weight Gain

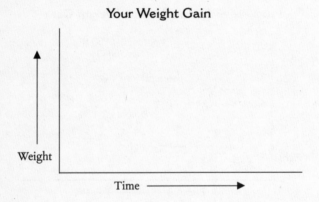

How do you feel when you look at your weight graph? Does it surprise you? Does it help you to better understand how life events may have affected your weight? One patient said that this exercise jolted her because for the first time she could clearly see why she had had such difficulties with her weight. Previously, she hadn't made the connection between her weight gain and the financial stress of her business, the worsening health of her aging mother, and the increasing time demands from her children. With a better understanding of the life events she had endured and their impact on her weight, she stopped blaming herself (and even began practicing forgiveness) and was ready to take charge of her weight and her life. This exercise helped another patient realize that her job promotion had moved her into an isolated social situation, which then resulted in consuming more comfort food and gaining weight. Seeking social support became as important a goal as weight loss itself. For yet another patient, it became clear that work had become his number one priority in life and it was time for him to shift gears and refocus on himself—and his health. If you want more information about how to determine the health risks associated with your weight, see the BMI table and "Know Your BMI" in Appendix A.

So if false weight is the extra weight adults gain while focusing on other life events, you may be asking what is one's authentic shape and, most important, how do you recover yours? Though you already have a general definition of authentic shape, only you can determine what it looks like, how it feels, and when you know you've reclaimed it. Here's how some patients have felt when they've recovered theirs:

"I feel energetic and I'm not tired all the time."
"I feel comfortable in my smaller clothes."
"I'm no longer embarrassed to shop for clothes."
"I take risks and try new things I never would have done before."
"I feel more in control of my weight and my life."
"I feel younger."
"I feel more alive and connected with people."
"I feel more sexually attractive."
"For once I feel people are not judging me by my weight."
"I can get down on the floor and play with my kids."
"I can climb stairs without feeling short of breath."
"I like what I see in the mirror."

Similar to these patients, you will probably find that recovering your authentic shape is not slimming down to your weight at age 18, nor is it about reaching some magical number on the bathroom scale. That's because your authentic shape takes into account your feelings and activities (in addition to your weight) and connects your mind and body like never before. Look over these statements again. Think about how you would feel if you could achieve some of these benefits. You see, another problem causing people to succumb to the pressures of scaling up syndrome has been a misunderstanding about how to accomplish weight loss. Because of conflicting information in the media, you are likely focusing on the wrong things and in the wrong ways. You probably go for the one-dimensional, quick "food fix" solution, which doesn't address the other key elements of scaling up syndrome such as how you move (or don't move) your body or how you cope with stress. As you will learn, if your weight loss tactics are not multidimensional and woven into and throughout the different aspects of your life, then these strategies are bound to fail. This means that your mind has to be connected to what your body is doing and vice versa. It's a method that works, and I'll show you how. But before you can learn how to scale down, I recommend that you better understand the factors (missing from most diet books) that caused you to scale up.

Scaling Up American Style

In the following sections, you'll learn how different life events can cause you to gain weight and how food, inactivity, and stress play varying roles depending on your particular stage of life. Since these life events are a part of your natural progression through adulthood, you may never have thought much about their relationship to your weight gain. Or like some of my patients if you have thought about it, maybe you blamed yourself. I will help you to identify the real culprit in scaling up syndrome—our unhealthy environment. And once you understand that you are not at fault, your battle to take back control of your weight will be halfway won.

The "Freshman 10"

Years ago, the weight teens gained when they went off to college was called the "freshman 10." Today, with fast-food restaurants on most campus street corners, it's called the "freshman 15." This time of life has its unique challenges, when autonomy and fitting in often prevail over focusing on one's personal eating and fitness behaviors. And whatever eating and activity patterns students bring with them from home can change drastically. So some students eat pizza late at night because that's what everyone else is doing— not because they're hungry. Others snack on candy while studying because their roommate keeps it around. Still others have trouble controlling food portions from their buffet-style dorm meals. Also round-the-clock availability of high-calorie, high-fat fast food offers students quick, good-tasting, and cheap meals. And value meals with supersize portions can be hard for anyone to resist—especially anyone on a tight budget. Experimenting with alcoholic beverages can also quickly add on the pounds. So begins one's experiences away from home with the socialization of eating and drinking.

Meanwhile, a college student's activity level may be changed from high school depending on whether or not the student walks to and from classes, has easy access to the campus exercise facility, or participates in sports. This is also a time when body image becomes more acute. And with the increase in eating disorders on college campuses, as some students are gaining weight, ironically others are starving themselves—and neither group is satisfied with their bodies. Social influences at this stage of life are so strong and pervasive that one can easily gain a few pounds here and a few there, and before long you leave college with excess pounds and some newly acquired life habits.

Career Gains

With each new stage of life, the challenges and social pressures change. The schedule and demands of work often begin to shape early adulthood eating, exercise, and coping patterns—and rarely toward health. Even the basic act of eating in the midst of a typical workday poses difficulties for many patients, who frequently complain about not finding time for lunch, having difficulty eating the right foods on the run, and having trouble resisting the temptations to snack throughout the workday. And with the availability of high-calorie and savory snacks in vending machines, at airport terminals, gas stations, and office supply stores, workday eating is typically unhealthy and contains more calories than the body can handle. Though we can control food brought into and left in our homes, we really have no control over food brought into the workplace, the number of vending machines that line our break rooms, or the types of fast food readily available by phone, fax, or E-mail.

> ➣ *Nibble on This* ➢
> Fifty percent of employed women and 40 percent of employed men surveyed by the National Restaurant Association felt they now have less time for lunch.

While temptations to overeat prevail for our collective workforce, our daily dependence on modern technology, those labor-saving devices such as elevators, escalators, E-mail, faxes, and computers keep us sedentary or sitting at our desks instead of moving our bodies. This trend has captured the attention of obesity expert Dr. Gary Foster of the University of Pennsylvania, who calls the growing number of computer addicts "mouse potatoes." Though the good news is that some couch potatoes have jumped off of their couches, the bad news is that they've landed in front of their monitors for hours on end. Patients are typically surprised at how productive and active their minds can be at work while their bodies remain idle. And though at first they can be resistant to adding any activities to their daily schedule, they become more receptive once they discover how small activities can add up over time to make a big difference.

> ⮞ *Nibble on This* ⮜
>
> According to Dr. William Haskell of Stanford University, using E-mail (for 5 minutes per workday hour) to talk to coworkers rather than walking to their offices has caused the average worker to gain a pound a year or 10 pounds in a decade.

You may also find that you are caught in a cycle of working hard and after work having the energy only to plop your body on the sofa and watch television. However, instead of energizing you, lying around often makes your body feel more tired. In an article in *Redbook*, stress expert Paul Wilson said "to unwind, many of us watch television programs that we're not particularly interested in, and spend much of our free time in a state of low-level boredom. But boredom is actually tension-inducing because it makes you feel as if you don't have control over your life." It's no wonder that patients soon realize they need to find new ways to lift their spirits and to energize both their mind and body.

Finding Family/Losing Self

Though everyone has his or her own story to tell, the common thread through most patients' stories is that they typically put family members' needs before their own. So some dieters continue to overeat rich restaurant food because that's what their husbands like, others stop cooking healthy foods because a family member hates vegetables, and yet others continue to keep unhealthy snack foods at home because that's what their children or grandchildren like. Still other patients relate that carpooling or a child's after-school activities quickly eat up time that could have been devoted to an exercise routine or to other personal needs. Subtly and oh so innocently, your best intentions toward weight loss may be thwarted by loved ones around you. And month after month, year after year, or even decade after decade, doing for everyone else first takes its toll.

Because the family caregiver has so much control over the health of the home environment, if this is your role, you need to understand how the pressures of scaling up syndrome make this responsibility more difficult than you might guess. Consider grocery shopping. In a society where time is limited, advertising budgets are high, and product choices are endless, it's easy to feel as if you're losing control at the supermarket. At a local grocery store, we recently counted 178 different kinds of boxed cereals, 100 different kinds of cookies, and 150 different types of salad dressings. Though most people like having choices, this seems just a bit excessive.

⇒ Nibble on This ⇐

By 4 P.M., 80 percent of grocery shoppers do not know what they're having for dinner that night.

While serious cooking is out for many busy families, assembling meals, ordering takeout, or dining out is in. Patients quickly learn that the more they order in and dine out, the less control they have over their diet. That's because food eaten away from home is generally higher in fat and saturated fat, and lower in fiber and calcium than is food prepared at home, according to the USDA's two-decade-long study of food intake. Many nutrition experts agree that fat is not the only culprit; portions also play a role, as the expected serving sizes in restaurants have grown to anywhere from two to four times the USDA's recommended portion size. What begins with a healthy longing to relax and treat ourselves can cause us to indulge and overeat.

> ⤳ *Nibble on This* ⤶
>
> The 64-ounce steak served at a popular Chicago steakhouse is sixteen times the USDA recommended portion size of 4 ounces.

Handling Ups and Downs

Good or bad—it's always something. It's interesting how for one person the stress that results from a divorce or from being laid off from work can result in a 15-pound weight gain while for another person it can mean losing 15 pounds. And for some people, happy times such as vacations or celebrations can affect weight gain just as easily as can sad times such as grieving over the loss of a loved one. It doesn't seem fair that handling both life's ups and its downs can affect scaling up syndrome. But since food is always on the guest list at both parties and funerals, it is just a part of our culture that we must accept.

A special birthday, a romantic anniversary, a religious holiday, or even a promotion can make you want to lay back, throw out all the rules, and just enjoy. And you should—within moderation. Holidays, especially between Thanksgiving and Christmas, are a time when many people find themselves gaining up to 5 to 10 pounds. All the seasonal holiday foods, snacks, parties, and leftovers are simply too much to handle. Other common pressures related to their weight gain are a death in the family, losing a business, a divorce, caring for an ill parent, or suffering from an illness oneself. The stress of these immediate and serious problems causes many people to eat poorly temporarily and drop their exercise routine, whereas others actually become clinically depressed. This is real life. An important part of this program is helping you to acknowledge your emotions and give yourself permission for these feelings, and to find healthier ways to calm yourself during these trying times. You can learn how to prepare for life's unexpected curveballs.

Having Unrealistic Ideals

As if it's not hard enough to gain control of your weight in the midst of real-life struggles and challenges, there's yet one more element to scaling up that cannot go unmentioned. The "unreal" images in magazines, in newspapers, on television, in movies, and on billboards pressure you to strive for a beauty ideal that is unattainable. Radiating success, happiness, and the good life that you are trying so hard to achieve, these images have a powerful influence on your subconscious mind. At the same time, advertisements for quick-fix diet products make weight loss look so easy. These messages feed on your vulnerability, support the notion that you are at fault for your weight problems, and can steer you down futile or dangerous dieting paths.

Since I frequently help patients to confront unrealistic beauty ideals, throughout the book I will help you too. Even if you don't currently relate to this problem, subconsciously these images can set you up for failure as you set a weight loss goal that's unachievable and unrealistic. So even if you lose the recommended 10–15 percent of your body weight, you're still not satisfied because it's just not enough.

> ➢ *Nibble on This* ➣
> The average height and weight of a model is 5'9" and 110 pounds (considered "underweight") while the average American woman is 5'4" and 142 pounds (at the upper limits of a healthy body weight).

Scaling Down

For most every scaling up pressure in this chapter, a corresponding strategy exists for scaling down. I have organized this book so that you will gently advance from point to point through these strategies. Some of you may be in the throes of a commercial weight loss program but are unhappy with the results. Others may have spent the last five years procrastinating about losing weight. Still others may have recently tried a high-protein, low-carbohydrate diet but know that it's not a healthy program to stay on for life. Wherever you are in your weight loss journey will be your beginning place. And by this time in the book, if you have stopped blaming yourself for your weight gain and have a better understanding of how scaling up syndrome has affected you, then you are ready to scale down.

Getting Started

To get you started, the three-week starter plan (see Appendix B) is the same one that I routinely give patients on their first visit. And without question, each and every patient who completes this plan returns a changed person: having a higher level of awareness and as a bonus, losing on average 5 pounds—though some patients lose from 10 to 16 pounds! As one patient commented after completing this three-week plan and losing 7½ pounds, "I felt as if I was making positive observations and changes without being on a diet."

In contrast to the rest of the book, which is very focused and personalized to your particular lifestyle patterns, this plan is more general. But it has grown into an essential program component that gives you practice reshaping your eating, exercise, and coping patterns in three different environments—home, work, and social. I call it the "3 × 3 program" because it focuses on 3 environments, 3 behaviors, in 3 weeks. Though you can expect to lose approximately 1 to 2 pounds each week, the focus of this plan is as much on the process of changing your lifestyle habits as on the resultant weight loss. I include a checklist at the end of each week to help you mark your progress.

Working through this 3 × 3 program will help you to lose weight and it will also deepen your self-awareness. For one, you will have a better understanding of how the pressures of scaling up syndrome play out in your life—at home, at work, and in social situations. Also, you will have a better understanding of your support persons and your saboteurs. Sharing your intentions with the right people sets you up for success. Then too you will be more aware of the roles eating, activity, and coping have when it comes to your weight. With this new understanding, you are ready to discover your diet personality and the path to your authentic shape.

■ ■ ■ ■ ■

Chapter 2

Discovering Your Diet Personality

Your personality embodies those attitudes, behaviors, habits, and emotions that distinguish you from others. These personal and social traits even affect the particular lifestyle you lead, especially as it relates to your weight. I have found that when people identify their diet personality profile—their unique combination of eating, exercise, and coping lifestyle patterns—they can successfully work with their profile to shed weight for good. If you don't get a handle on your diet personality, these patterns slowly creep back into your life and reverse your success.

> ⪼ *Nibble on This* ⪻
>
> "Most people underestimate their power to change and grow. They believe that yesterday's pattern must be tomorrow's."
>
> —DR. NATHANIEL BRANDON, *THE SIX PILLARS OF SELF-ESTEEM*

Diet Personality Quiz

To help you to identify your diet personality profile, please complete the following Diet Personality Quiz by reading each statement and then placing a check in the column that best reflects your level of agreement with the statement. Take care to record how you currently act and feel (not how you may have acted or felt some time in the past).

Diet Personality Quiz

Eating Inventory	Agree on Occasion or Disagree 0	Agree Much of the Time 1	Agree Most of the Time 2	Agree All of the Time 3
1. I do not have consistent meal patterns from one day to the next.		✓		
2. I rarely take the time to plan my meals.			✓	
3. I'm rarely hungry in the morning.				✓
4. I often skip breakfast.				✓
5. I eat little during the day and am most hungry at night.	✓			
6. I eat most of my food in the evening, at dinner and after.			✓	✓
7. Most meals are takeout or eaten in restaurants.		✓		
8. I eat a fast-food meal on most days of the week.		✓		
9. I rarely eat fresh foods or home-cooked meals.		✓		
10. I eat much more processed snack foods than fresh ones.			✓	
11. Fruits and vegetables are my least favorite foods.	✓			
12. I know I should be eating more fruits and vegetables than I am.	✓			
13. Given a choice, I seldom choose fruits and vegetables.		✓		
14. Hungry or not, I snack on foods throughout the day.	✓	✓		
15. Hungry or not, I snack on foods at home.		✓		
16. Hungry or not, I snack on foods brought into the workplace.	✓			
17. My snacking directly relates to the presence of food around me.		✓		
18. I have difficulty controlling my portion sizes.			✓	
19. I overeat at buffets.				✓
20. I never feel full until it's too late.				✓

21. Eating is always a battle between what I want to eat and what I think I should eat.		✓		
22. If I "cheat" on my diet, I feel guilty afterward.	✓			
23. I have two eating styles: the "good" one I show in public and the "bad" one I do in private.	✓			

Activity Inventory

24. I do not like to exercise.	✓			
25. I am not an athletic person.	✓			
26. Being physically active has never been one of my priorities.		✓		
27. I'm too embarrassed by my body to go to a gym.	✓			
28. I think others are always looking at how big and out of shape I am.	✓			
29. My heightened awareness of other people's and my own body size and shape prevents me from exercising.	✓			
30. My attitude about exercising is neither good nor bad.		✓		
31. I don't know the first thing about how to get started with an exercise program.	✓			
32. I have never exercised and will need direction.	✓			
33. I alternate between being sedentary and working out excessively.		✓		
34. If I can't do my full workout, I typically do nothing at all.	✓			
35. Once my week-to-week exercise routine is interrupted, I find it very hard to get back on track.		✓		
36. I do exercise regularly, but I'm in a rut.	✓			
37. I have been doing the same workout for the past 3 months or more.	✓			
38. I'm bored with my exercise routine.		✓		

Activity Inventory *(cont.)*	Agree on Occasion or Disagree 0	Agree Much of the Time 1	Agree Most of the Time 2	Agree All of the Time 3
39. I don't usually vary the intensity, duration, or frequency of my workout from session to session.			✓	
40. I have physical limitations that make it difficult for me to be active.	✓			
41. I limit my exercise because I fear injury or stress on my heart.	✓			
42. It hurts when I exercise.	✓			
43. Despite trying, I can't seem to fit exercise into my hectic schedule.			✓	
44. I want to exercise but have little time to devote to being more active.			✓	
Coping Inventory				
45. I find myself eating instead of expressing my emotions.	✓			
46. I have a hard time sharing my feelings with friends and family.	✓			
47. Food is my trusted friend and comfort source.	✓			
48. I often eat when I'm stressed, lonely, anxious, or depressed.		✓		
49. I feel ashamed of my body.	✓			
50. Being embarrassed about my weight has impaired my social life.	✓			
51. I want to cry when I think about my weight.	✓			
52. Negative self-talk makes me my own worst enemy.	✓			
53. I know I need to lose weight but can never seem to get started.			✓	
54. I spend more time thinking about what I need to do to lose weight than actually doing something about it.			✓	
55. I do a lot to help others but not enough to help myself.	✓	✓		

56. I have a hard time asking others for help.	✓			
57. I often put myself last on my to-do list.	✓			
58. My pace of life is out of control, and I don't know how to slow it down.	✓			
59. I feel like I'm juggling too many things at once and have little time for myself.	✓	✓		
60. My mind is often on the next task before I complete the first one.		✓		
61. I am usually doubtful that a new weight loss program will work for me.		✓		
62. I want to lose weight, but I have yet to find someone who can help me.	✓			
63. I've tried everything to lose weight and nothing ever works.	✓			
64. High expectations cause me to feel disappointed even when I'm making progress.	✓			
65. I've had a high degree of success in my work and home life and expect the same of my weight loss.			✓	
66. I have problems setting realistic weight loss goals for myself.	✓			

Diet Personality Profile

To score your diet personality quiz, use the Diet Personality Key on pages 20–22 and complete the following:

1. First, fill in your scores for Identifying Statements 1–66 (using the listed scoring criteria).
2. Next, fill in your Total Scores for each pattern, by adding together the scores of the Identifying Statements.
3. Now calculate and record your Percentage Scores for each pattern by dividing the total score by the listed maximum pattern points possible.

For example, in the Sample Diet Personality Key on pages 22–24, the unguided grazer total score was 0. So 0 ÷ by 6 (the maximum points possible for the unguided grazer) = a percentage score of 0. The total score for the fruitless feaster was 6. So 6 ÷ by 9 (the maximum points possible for the fruitless feaster) = a percentage score of .67 or 67%.

Diet Personality Key

Pattern Names	Identifying Statements	Statement Scores	Total Scores	Percentage Scores
		Score your responses: **0**: Agree on occasion or disagree **1**: Agree much of the time **2**: Agree most of the time **3**: Agree all the time	Add up the individual statement scores.	Divide total score by the listed maximum pattern points possible.
Eating Patterns				
Unguided Grazer	1 2	1 2		Total Score ÷ 6 = 0.50
Nighttime Nibbler	3 4 5 6	3 3 0 2		Total Score ÷ 12 = .66
Convenient Consumer	7 8 9 10	1 1 1 2		Total Score ÷ 12 = .42
Fruitless Feaster	11 12 13	0 0 1		Total Score ÷ 9 = .11
Mindless Muncher	14 15 16 17	0 1 0 1		Total Score ÷ 12 = .17
Hearty Portioner	18 19 20	2 3 3		Total Score ÷ 9 = .89
Deprived Sneaker	21 22 23	1 0 0		Total Score ÷ 9 = .11

Diet Personality Key *(cont.)*

Exercise Patterns				
Hate-to-Move Struggler	24 25 26	0 0 1		Total Score ÷ 9 = .11
Self-Conscious Hider	27 28 29	0 0 0		Total Score ÷ 9 = 0
Inexperienced Novice	30 31 32	1 0 0		Total Score ÷ 9 = .11
All-or-Nothing Doer	33 34 35	1 0 1		Total Score ÷ 9 = .22
Set-Routine Repeater	36 37 38 39	0 0 1 2		Total Score ÷ 12 = .25
Aches-and-Pains Sufferer	40 41 42	0 0 0		Total Score ÷ 9 =
No-Time-to-Exercise Protester	43 44	2 2		Total Score ÷ 6 = 67
Coping Patterns				
Emotional Stuffer	45 46 47 48	0 0 0 1		Total Score ÷ 12 = 0.08
Low-Self-Esteem Sufferer	49 50 51 52	0 0 0 0		Total Score ÷ 12 = 0
Persistent Procrastinator	53 54	2 2		Total Score ÷ 6 = .67
Can't-Say-No Pleaser	55 56 57	0 0 0		Total Score ÷ 9 = 0
Fast Pacer	58 59 60	0 0 1		Total Score ÷ 9 = 0.11

Diet Personality Key *(cont.)*

Coping Patterns				
Pessimistic Thinker	61 62 63	_1_ _0_ _0_		Total Score ÷ 9 = _0.11_
Unrealistic Achiever	64 65 66	_0_ _2_ _0_		Total Score ÷ 9 = _0.22_

Sample Diet Personality Key

Pattern Names	Identifying Statements	Statement Scores	Total Scores	Percentage Scores
		Score your responses: 0: Agree on occasion or disagree 1: Agree much of the time 2: Agree most of the time 3: Agree all the time	Add up the individual statement scores.	Divide total score by the listed maximum pattern points possible.
Eating Patterns				
Unguided Grazer	1 2	0 0	0	Total Score (0) ÷ 6 = **0**
Nighttime Nibbler	3 4 5 6	0 0 0 0	0	Total Score (0) ÷ 12 = **0**
Convenient Consumer	7 8 9 10	0 0 0 2	2	Total Score (2) ÷ 12 = **.17 or 17%**
Fruitless Feaster	11 12 13	2 2 2	6	Total Score (6) ÷ 9 = **.67 or 67%**
Mindless Muncher	14 15 16 17	0 1 0 1	2	Total Score (2) ÷ 12 = **.17 or 17%**

Sample Diet Personality Key *(cont.)*

Hearty Portioner	18 19 20	3 2 2	7	Total Score (7) ÷ 9 = **.78 or 78%**
Deprived Sneaker	21 22 23	0 0 0	0	Total Score (0) ÷ 9 = **0**
Exercise Patterns				
Hate-to-Move Struggler	24 25 26	1 1 0	2	Total Score (2) ÷ 9 = **.22 or 22%**
Self-Conscious Hider	27 28 29	3 2 2	7	Total Score (7) ÷ 9 = .78 or 78%
Inexperienced Novice	30 31 32	0 0 0	0	Total Score (0) ÷ 9 = **0**
All-or-Nothing Doer	33 34 35	0 0 0	0	Total Score (0) ÷ 9 = **0**
Set-Routine Repeater	36 37 38 39	0 0 0 0	0	Total Score (0) ÷ 12 = **0**
Aches-and Pains Sufferer	40 41 42	0 0 0	0	Total Score (0) ÷ 9 = **0**
No-Time-to-Exercise Protester	43 44	3 2	5	Total Score (5) ÷ 6 = **.83 or 83%**
Coping Patterns				
Emotional Stuffer	45 46 47 48	0 0 0 1	1	Total Score (1) ÷ 12 = **.08 or 8%**
Low-Self-Esteem Sufferer	49 50 51 52	0 0 0 0	0	Total Score (0) ÷ 12 = **0**

Sample Diet Personality Key *(cont.)*

Coping Patterns				
Persistent Procrastinator	53 54	2 3	5	Total Score (5) ÷ 6 = **.83 or 83%**
Can't-Say-No 9 Pleaser	55 56 57	2 2 3	7	Total Score (7) ÷ = **.78 or 78%**
Fast Pacer	58 59 60	0 0 0	0	Total Score (0) ÷ 9 = **0**
Pessimistic Thinker	61 62 63	0 1 0	1	Total Score (1) ÷ 9 = **.11 or 11%**
Unrealistic Achiever	64 65 66	2 1 2	5	Total Score (5) ÷ 9 = **.56 or 56%**

Patients in my program also benefit from seeing their actual pattern score distribution, as shown in the following sample eating, exercise, and coping pattern profile graphs. You'll see that the height of each pattern bar matches the pattern's percentage score (from the previous sample). For example, the bar for the unrealistic achiever extends to its percentage score level of .56 or 56%. If this interests you, take a few minutes to draw bars on the blank profile graphs to match your pattern scores. Alternatively, just skip over the profile graphs and continue on page 27.

Sample Diet Personality Profile

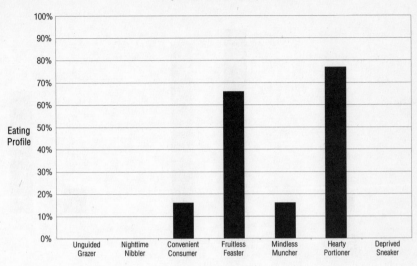

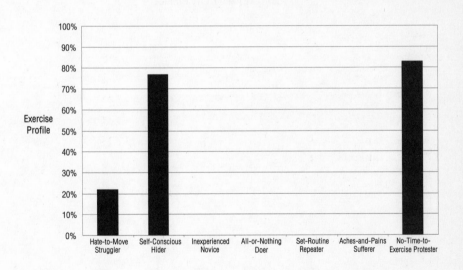

Dr. Kushner's Personality Type Diet

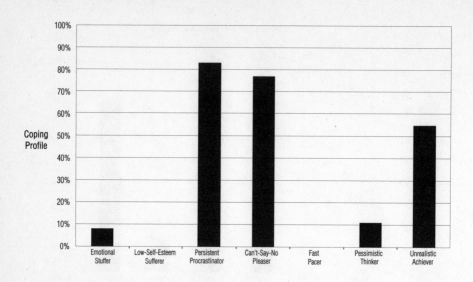

Coping Profile

Emotional Stuffer · Low-Self-Esteem Sufferer · Persistent Procrastinator · Can't-Say-No Pleaser · Fast Pacer · Pessimistic Thinker · Unrealistic Achiever

Your Diet Personality Profiles

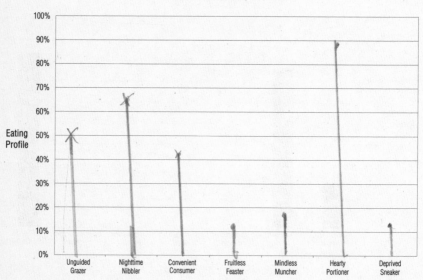

Eating Profile

Unguided Grazer · Nighttime Nibbler · Convenient Consumer · Fruitless Feaster · Mindless Muncher · Hearty Portioner · Deprived Sneaker

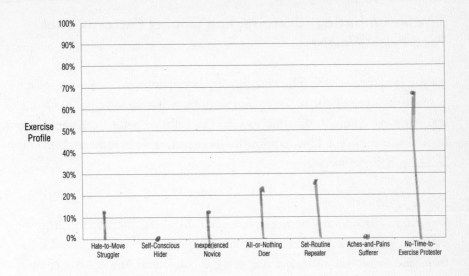

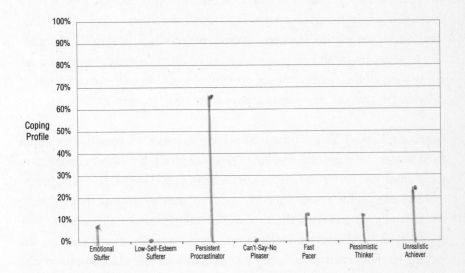

Your pattern percentage scores (and the visual graphs if you completed them) form your overall diet personality profile, which personalizes my weight loss program to you and your particular lifestyle. As one patient said after calculating her pattern percentage scores, "Dr. Kushner, you've really pegged me." This motivated her because she felt as if someone finally understood her. Now it's time for you to read the pattern descriptions (paying special attention to the highest scores or the predominant ones from your profiles) to see if I've pegged you too.

The Seven Eating, Exercise, and Coping Patterns That Feed False Weight

As you read through the following pattern descriptions, you will start seeing yourself in some of them. Take comfort in knowing that you are not alone and it's more common than not to relate to multiple patterns. Later in the book, I will show you how to prioritize these patterns and reshape them one by one to achieve success.

Eating Patterns

Unguided Grazer. Eating occurs anytime and anywhere since food is an afterthought. Without any structure or planning, your diet varies tremendously from one day to the next. But one thing is consistent: You usually choose foods that are convenient and readily accessible. Also, because food is often consumed while the grazer attends to other activities—such as driving, working, or surfing the Internet—you frequently lack a conscious connection to your hunger and eat past your point of satiety. Consequently, you are not getting all the right nutrients, are probably eating excessive amounts of calories, fat, and salt, and portions vary from small to oversized.

Nighttime Nibbler. You consume 50 percent or more of your daily calories from dinner and nighttime snacking. You may go all day without eating anything since you aren't hungry or are denying your hunger. Some nighttime nibblers simply don't make time to eat during the day because they put their work, family, or travel schedules ahead of taking care of themselves. This approach always backfires. By sundown, they are ravenous and end up consuming far more calories than they intended. Dinner often blends into continual trips to the kitchen for repeated snacking that ends only by falling asleep. The next morning, full of remorse, you swear off food only to find yourself racing to the fridge at the end of the workday. Since you consume most of your calories when your metabolism is slowest, your excess calories are more likely to turn into fat.

Convenient Consumer. A diet of convenience, packaged, bagged, microwaveable, and frozen foods are the staples of your diet. All foods listed in your diet diary bear a brand name that is posted on the box, menu, or restaurant chain.

There are very few (if any) fresh foods or home-cooked meals. The problem with this dietary pattern is that these foods are generally higher in fat, sodium, and calories and lower in fiber than fresh foods cooked at home. Also, many in this camp eat within a small range of foods—perhaps McDonald's on Mondays, Taco Bell on Tuesdays, and Wendy's on Wednesdays—and suffer from a lack of nutritional variety.

Fruitless Feaster. You enjoy a plain meat and potatoes menu. With the exception of a daily glass of orange juice and an occasional apple or banana, the feaster sticks to proteins, breads, pastas, fats, and desserts. According to the most recent population study, only 20 percent of Americans consume a daily serving of fresh fruits and vegetables. The goal is to consume 5 or more servings every day of these great cancer and heart disease fighters. Feasters miss out on the vitamins, minerals, fiber, and phytonutrients of these powerful foods, which are low calorie to boot.

Mindless Muncher. You are committed to eating 3 meals a day (a good start). However, there is also snacking going on throughout the day and night— whether hungry or not. Some people snack out of a fear of getting hungry. Others snack to fight boredom or to take a break in the middle of the day. Still others cannot pass up a plate or package of food, a vending machine, or a snack shop— whether at home, the workplace, their place of worship, a social outing, or running errands. Simply the sight or smell of any food triggers their compulsion to eat. The problem is that mindless eating causes you to eat excess calories while not really tasting or enjoying your food.

Hearty Portioner. You may feel that your stomach is a bottomless pit and you eat oversized portions in an effort to fill it. Some hearty portioners overindulge on unhealthy foods, while others overeat healthy ones. In both cases, they eat quickly, their weight is climbing steadily, and they feel powerless to change the pattern. With a food diary generally showing an intake that is two to five times the norm, you were probably raised as a member of the "clean your plate club." You are usually stuffed after eating, feel ashamed of your gluttony, and swear you won't overeat again—until the next time. You may also suffer from indigestion, heartburn, or reflux after meals, along with sluggishness and fatigue.

Deprived Sneaker. You eat a strict diet of "good" foods only to fall off the wagon and overeat "bad" foods. Here's what this pattern looks like in action: Instead of eating a small slice of that chocolate cake, you choose fat-free cookies; but despite eating eight cookies, you still feel deprived of what you really wanted—the chocolate cake. Having what you really wanted from the beginning would have saved you many calories and emotional suffering. For the deprived sneaker, food is always a battle between eating "good" foods in public that you don't always enjoy and sneaking anything "bad" in private that tastes good but makes you feel guilty. You never feel satisfied.

Exercise Patterns

Hate-to-Move Struggler. Even when younger, you were never encouraged to be physically active, didn't like to sweat, and typically didn't have the coordination to excel in sports. You may even sadly recall embarrassing experiences such as being picked last on gym teams or being laughed at by peers. As you got on with your life, inactivity became even more acceptable, which reinforced your disregard for physical exercise.

Self-Conscious Hider. You feel socially phobic about exercising in public. Just the thought of being with other people in an enclosed exercise space may keep you out of the gym. Because you have a hyperawareness of your own body compared to other people's body sizes (especially when wearing tight workout clothes and when jumping around), you are not able to relax your mind or body long enough to enjoy any group exercise experience.

Inexperienced Novice. Without prior bad or good attitudes about exercise, the life of the inexperienced novice has never been physically active. Either your job never demanded much physical activity or you never played sports. You simply don't know how to exercise.

All-or-Nothing Doer. This is the weekend warrior who after a sedentary workweek spends hours pounding the pavement or intensely working out at the gym. Or maybe you join a health club and intensely work out 4 to 5 days a week for months and then, because something gets in your way (such as an injury, a work project, or stress at home), you end up being sedentary for months on end. The all-or-nothing doer is typically a goal-oriented, driven person whose all-or-nothing characteristics reflect a personality trait seen also at work and home. What you don't realize is that inconsistent exercise makes you more injury-prone.

Set-Routine Repeater. You are typically frustrated about not losing more weight because you already exercise regularly. On questioning however, it is apparent that you've been doing a fixed exercise routine—such as walking on the treadmill at the same speed for the same duration or maybe walking outside 3 times a week for a half hour each time. By staying at your comfortable pace and not challenging your body, your body becomes so efficient in what it's doing that you don't get the same benefit. And many repeaters also become bored.

Aches-and-Pains Sufferer. You either already have an established medical problem or injury that impairs your ability to exercise (arthritis with achy joints, a bad back, foot or arm problems, heart disease), or you worry that exercise may bring on a heart attack or injury since you feel so out of shape. Differing attitudes are also important, as one sufferer may be truly frustrated and angry she can't exercise, while someone else may develop a resistance or defiance to exercise—having developed a "yes, but" attitude.

No-Time-to-Exercise Protester. You are busy at work and home and the local community. You're likely to be very frustrated because you know you need to exercise but can't seem to squeeze it into your hectic schedule.

Coping Patterns

Emotional Stuffer. You typically use food as comfort. Since food never talks back, it becomes your trusted and reliable friend when stressed, anxious, lonely, or depressed. No matter how bad things get, food can always make you feel better.

Low Self-Esteem Sufferer. You are your own worst enemy, as you frequently engage in negative self-talk. Feeling ashamed of your body also impairs your social life and feelings of self-worth. When you look in the mirror you may overemphasize particular body parts, such as your hips or thighs. Having trouble separating your body image from your self-esteem affects your social skills, relationships, and even day-to-day decision making.

Persistent Procrastinator. You know the importance of losing weight and frequently verbalize this important priority. But you never seem to make it happen because something else (another work deadline or family responsibility) always gets in the way. You may be anxious and fearful about starting (and possibly failing) another program. You're also frustrated and tired of saying you'll get to it next week, when next week never seems to come.

Can't-Say-No Pleaser. You are a good-natured person who has a strong sense of responsibility and commitment to your family, coworkers, and volunteer causes. What you lack, however, is a commitment or know-how about how to take care of your own health needs at the same time. You simply can't say no, and people take advantage of this.

Fast Pacer. You are an expert at multitasking and juggling. But you move so fast through life that your mind doesn't know what your body is doing and vice versa. You may eat so fast that you don't really taste the food, or you may be doing so much that you have no time to think or plan ways to improve your lifestyle. Do you talk on the cell phone while walking down the street, driving, dining, or even during doctor appointments? You may think you're listening but often your mind is elsewhere. You typically feel frazzled and have trouble relaxing.

Pessimistic Thinker. You say you've tried everything and nothing works. In addition to feeling hopeless, you develop the self-defeating attitude that no one can help you. If others offer help, you may get angry with them—pushing help away instead of welcoming it. Instead of looking at life events as challenges and opportunities, you look at them as hurdles and barriers.

Unrealistic Achiever. You have achieved a high degree of success in your work and home life—and you expect the same level of success with your weight. But regardless of the progress you make, it's never enough. Your high expectations leave you feeling frustrated and discouraged.

How You Compare

In case you're wondering how your pattern scores compare with those of other dieters, I'd like to share with you my research study results. In 2001, I asked one hundred new patients participating in my weight management program at Northwestern Memorial Hospital to fill out the diet personality quiz. These were individuals who had generally struggled with their weight for years and were looking for real answers. They were a variety of ethnicities, ranged in age from 22 to 62 and weighed from 121 to 514 pounds. There were 83 women and 17 men.

It was interesting to note how strongly these patients identified with the same eating, exercise, and coping lifestyle pattern descriptions that you just read. Among these patients, the average number of eating, exercise, and coping patterns was 3 eating, 3 exercise, and 4 coping patterns (based on a threshold of .33 or above as being a significant pattern). As you can see in the table below, those patients with fewer pounds to lose had a lower number of significant patterns than those with more pounds to lose. That didn't surprise me; you would expect that the more overweight someone is, the more symptoms (or symptom patterns, in this case) he or she has.

Pattern Relationships

Eating Patterns	Exercise Patterns	Coping Patterns	Patients with 5–35 Pounds to Lose	Patients with 35–60 Pounds to Lose
98% related to them	95% related to them	99% related to them	On average, had 2 eating, 2 exercise, and 2–3 coping patterns	On average, had 3 eating, 3 exercise, and 4 coping patterns

Of course, your total number of significant patterns may fall below or above the averages. And you can expect that the more sensitive you are to the influences of scaling up syndrome, the higher your total number of patterns will be. What's most important, however, is not the number of patterns you have but which ones in each category have the highest scores, since these are the areas you'll want to focus on.

Prioritize Patterns

Now that you've identified your eating, exercise, and coping pattern scores, you need to prioritize them. Most of my patients want to tackle their eating profile first—which is fine with me, since this has the greatest effect on weight loss. Once patients are losing weight and feeling successful, they're usually more motivated to work on their exercise and then coping profiles. The only time patients deviate from this is when their coping patterns are interfering with their ability to focus on their eating or exercise patterns. For example, one woman was such a persistent procrastinator that she had trouble getting started tackling her nighttime nibbling pattern. For her, working first on her key coping pattern gave her the strategies she needed to stop procrastinating and take action. If you're motivated and ready to start with your eating patterns first, give them a try. If a coping pattern starts interfering with your success, then feel free to switch gears.

Once you determine the profile (eating, exercise, or coping) to start with, you need to choose which pattern in that category you want to undertake first. You should find one of the following three methods helpful.

- Look at your pattern scores or visual graph, starting with the pattern that has the highest score, and then work your way down to the one with the next highest score, and so on. Here, the most predominant patterns always take precedence and the less prominent patterns are left for fine-tuning your weight loss.
- Tackle what you perceive to be the easiest pattern to change or the one you can implement almost immediately. For example, if you are a fruitless feaster, immediately start adding fruit and vegetables to your meals and snacks.
- Select a pattern you think is most important to your long-term weight control. For example, it is difficult for pessimistic thinkers to stick to new eating and exercise behaviors without a positive mind-set.

Whichever method you choose will be right for you. The important thing is that you pick one of them and get started. It's up to you how long you spend on each pattern. For one person, 1 to 2 weeks may be enough, but another may need 3 weeks. Don't worry if it takes longer to integrate some strategies into your life—just think progress, not perfection. You'll know you're ready to tackle another pattern when you start feeling comfortable with your changing attitudes and behaviors. Do take care not to rush—you want to be able to adapt to these changes without feeling overwhelmed.

Use Tools to Build Success

Now that you have an idea of which patterns you want to work on, how do you actually change your profiles and build success in the process? After a lifetime of eating, moving, and coping in ways that feel comfortable and seemingly natural, it's important to use tools to help you move forward. Each of the twenty-one lifestyle patterns in Chapters 3, 4, and 5 contains a unique treatment approach with its own set of tools called Weight Busters and Success Boosters. In addition, the following self-monitoring tools will help you stay on track by keeping you accountable to the one person who most wants you to succeed—you.

The first tool I universally recommend to all my patients (because it's been proved to shape and support behavior change) is the simple act of writing down or tracking the behaviors you want to change. Keeping a diary (or as my male patients call it a "journal") works because:

- it transforms your behaviors from being unconscious (mindless) to conscious (mindful). It increases awareness of what you are doing.
- it shows that you're serious.
- it reinforces the changes you need to make (for example, if you're a fruitless feaster, fruits and vegetables need to show up in your diary).
- it introduces the concept of planning as you start to think before you eat, or make time for exercising.
- it is therapeutic. People eat less when they know they will be recording their intake.

Many patients initially resist any kind of record keeping because they think it's too much work. But I recommend that they give it a try, even for 2 or 3 days. And patients who keep diaries end up losing more weight than patients who don't because even in the midst of a busy day, it helps them focus on their behaviors and feelings. It reminds them to pay attention and that their self-care is worth it. And most important, it reinforces their intended changes, keeping them in control.

Since the secret of successful, sustainable weight loss is to start with where you are and build from there, I recommend that at the beginning of this program you record at least 2 workdays and 1 weekend day (preferably consecutive) so that you can see if your habits vary with schedule and surroundings. Then periodically throughout the program (weekly and then monthly), you may find it helpful to refer back to this tool and use it as a barometer of how you're doing.

> *Nibble on This* <

If you previously tried a diet program that immediately started with a menu plan or asked you to eliminate entire food groups without first taking into consideration your eating patterns, lifestyle, and personal triggers, it most likely failed.

Here's how to get the most benefit from your daily Food, Mood, and Movement Diary (see the following blank and sample diaries). Starting first thing in the morning, record *when* you eat or drink, *what* you eat or drink, *how much* you eat or drink (the portion size using household measurements when possible, or an estimate), *where* you eat or drink, *why* you eat or drink (any associated emotional triggers such as sadness, loneliness, or anxiety, or activity-related triggers such as an argument with your spouse or a conflict at work, or an environmental trigger such as driving by a fast-food restaurant or walking by the kitchen), and *how hungry* you were before eating and drinking (on a scale of 0–4). At the bottom of the diary, record any planned activities or exercises that you performed.

Food, Mood, and Movement Diary

When? Time	What and How Much? Food/Beverage Portion Size	Where? Home/Work/ Car/Dining Out	Why? Associated Triggers: Stimuli, Emotions, Activities	How Hungry? (0—not hungry, 4—starving)

10-minute planned activity/exercise

Place check mark in box and document type of activity completed on the line. Each box represents 10 minutes of activity or exercise, signifying that activities can be broken up into manageable blocks of time.

☐ _____   ☐ _____
☐ _____   ☐ _____
☐ _____   ☐ _____
☐ _____   ☐ _____

Sample Food, Mood, and Movement Diary

When? Time	What and How Much? Food/Beverage Portion Size	Where? Home/Work/ Car/Dining Out	Why? Associated Triggers: Stimuli, Emotions, Activities	How Hungry? (0—not hungry, 4—starving)
6:00 A.M.	2 toaster waffles 1 bagel and cream cheese 1 banana 1 cup 2% milk 3 cups black coffee	Home (standing in kitchen, getting kids off to school)	Routine breakfast	3

Sample Food, Mood, and Movement Diary

When? Time	What and How Much? Food/Beverage Portion Size	Where? Home/Work/ Car/Dining Out	Why? Associated Triggers: Stimuli, Emotions, Activities	How Hungry? (0—not hungry, 4—starving)
7:30 A.M.	Doughnut 1 cup coffee	Office meeting (sitting at table)	Business meeting (vendor brought in donuts)	0
Noon	Tuna salad sandwich Potato chips, 1 bag 1 cookie 1 12-oz. Diet Coke	Cafeteria at work	Routine lunch	3
3:00 P.M.	1 chocolate candy bar 1 12-oz. Diet coke	Work (standing in break room)	Took bathroom break and passed vending machine on the way back to my desk	0
6:00 P.M.	Pizza with pepperoni, 3 slices 2 cups tossed salad 1 gingersnap cookie	Home (sitting with family at dinner table)	Didn't have time to prepare dinner	4
9:30 P.M.	1 large bowl Ben and Jerry's ice cream 2 cookies	Home (standing at kitchen counter)	Making kids' lunches for school tomorrow	0

10-minute planned activity/exercise
Place check mark in box and document type of activity completed on the line. Each box represents 10 minutes of activity or exercise, signifying that activities can be broken up into manageable blocks of time. This patient took a 10-minute walk at lunch and a 30-minute walk after dinner (40 minutes total).

☑ walk during lunch break _____   ☐ _____
☑ walk after dinner _____   ☐ _____
☑ walk after dinner _____   ☐ _____
☑ walk after dinner _____   ☐ _____

For best results, make these recordings "real time"—that is while you are eating rather than at the end of the day when your recording accuracy is bound to diminish. Alternatively, write down what you are planning to eat *before* you eat it. This gives you a chance to think twice about the ice cream, muffin, or third slice of pizza. The more you relax and have fun with this activity, the more you will learn about yourself, your relationship with food, and the impact of your environment.

I recommend that you use a similar food, mood, and movement diary. Instead of purchasing a special journal, simply copy these columns and headings inside a small, spiral notebook that you can keep at hand as your running log. Or make copies of the blank diary. To get the most benefit from this diary, you need to be able to compare the portions of food you record with recommended portion sizes. Though my patients often find food labels to be the best method for estimating their food portions, I'm giving you other ones as well. When you're in a restaurant or at a party and need to eyeball portions, try using the Quick Method to Estimate Portions. At home, you may find that the specific measurements in the Standard Serving Sizes table (or food labels) are more helpful—whatever method works best for you to get an accurate measure of your current consumption and to begin to calibrate your eye to healthy portion sizes.

Quick Method to Estimate Portions

Grain Group
1 serving = a slice of bread the size of a cassette tape
2 servings = a bagel the size of a hockey puck
1 serving = a large handful of cereal
1 serving = cooked cereal, rice, or pasta the size of a cupcake wrapper

Vegetable Group
1 serving = raw leafy vegetables equivalent to 4 outer romaine or iceberg leaves
1 serving = other vegetables, cooked or raw, the size of a small fist
2 servings = a medium potato the size of a computer mouse

Fruit Group
1 serving = a medium apple, orange, pear, or peach the size of a tennis ball
2 servings = chopped, cooked, or canned fruit the size of a baseball

Milk, Yogurt, and Cheese Group
1 serving = natural cheese the size of a 9-volt battery
1 serving milk = 1 cup

Meat, Poultry, Fish, Dry Beans, & Nuts Group
1 serving = cooked lean meat, fish, or poultry the size of a deck of cards
1 serving = peanut butter the size of a Ping-Pong ball
1 serving = a small handful of nuts or seeds

Source: ADA, *The Essential Guide to Nutrition & the Foods We Eat,* 1999.

Standard Serving Sizes

1 Serving from Breads, Cereals, Pasta, and Starchy Vegetables*	1 Serving from Vegetables*	1 Serving from Fruits*	1 Serving from Low-Fat Milk Products*	1 Serving from Meat, Fish, and Poultry*	1 Serving from Fats and Oils*
1 slice bread or ½ bagel or ½ English muffin	½ cup cooked or raw vegetable	1 whole piece of fruit such as medium apple, banana, or orange or 1 melon wedge or ½ cup berries	1 cup fat-free or 1% milk or 1 cup soy-based beverage with added calcium	3 ounces cooked (or 4 ounces raw) lean meat or poultry (2 thin slices roast beef, ½ chicken breast, or skinless chicken leg with thigh)	1 tsp. canola, corn, safflower, sesame, soybean, sunflower, or olive oil or regular margarine (no more than 2 grams of saturated fat per tablespoon)
½ cup hot cereal or 1 ounce ready-to-eat cereal (1 cup flaked cereal or ¼ cup nugget or bud-type cereal)	1 cup raw leafy vegetables	¾ cup fruit juice	1 cup nonfat or low-fat yogurt	3 ounces cooked (or 4 ounces raw) salmon, sardines, albacore tuna, herring, lake trout	1 tablespoon salad dressing or 2 teaspoons mayonnaise (with no more than 1 gram of saturated fat per tablespoon)
½ cup cooked rice or pasta	¾ cup vegetable juice	½ cup chopped, cooked, or canned fruit	½ cup low-fat cottage cheese	2½-ounce soyburger	2 teaspoons peanut butter** or 3 teaspoons nuts or seeds
¼–½ cup starchy vegetables (potatoes, corn, green peas, lima beans,*** winter squash, sweet potatoes, yams)	1 medium tomato or 5 cherry tomatoes	¼ cup dried fruit	1 ounce low-fat cheese (natural or processed cheeses with no more than 3 grams of fat and no more than 2 grams of saturated fat per ounce)	1 cup cooked beans, peas, or lentils*** or 3 ounces of tofu or 2 tablespoons peanut butter or ⅓ cup nuts or ¼ cup seeds**	⅛ medium avocado
1 four-inch pita bread or 1 seven-inch tortilla	1 cup vegetable soup	½ medium mango or ¼ medium papaya	½ cup fat-free or low-fat ice cream or frozen yogurt (no more than 3 grams of fat per ½-cup serving)	Eggs are no longer included with meat group because of their high cholesterol content of 213 mg. per yolk. Limit egg yolks to 3–4 per week. Egg whites or cholesterol-free egg substitutes can be used freely in cooking.	10 small or 5 large olives

Source: Adapted from American Heart Association 2000 Dietary Guidelines and the USDA.

Recommended number of servings per day: grains: 6–9; vegetables: 3–4; fruits: 2–3; dairy: 2–3; protein: 2–3; fat: no more than 5. The lower range of numbers correspond to a 1,600 calorie diet.

**Peanut butter, nuts, and seeds are all sources of both protein and fat.

***Beans can be counted as a serving of vegetables or meat, not both.

As you tackle your patterns in the next three chapters, keep in mind that being successful doesn't mean that you will attain 100 percent perfection for each and every pattern. Taking a few steps forward and a few back is an expected part of the behavior change process. Be flexible. Sometimes you may be up for working on multiple patterns, and other times one pattern will be more than enough. It's also entirely acceptable to address a particular pattern weeks or even months into the program. As long as you are making progress with any of the patterns, you are doing fine.

Chapter 3

Shaping Your Eating Personality

■ ■ ■ ■ O nce you identify your eating patterns, you'll see your true problem areas in stark relief. With this new self-awareness, you'll become more focused and ready to start a weight loss program that's finally grounded in your life. The strategies that follow directly address the influences of scaling up syndrome that have caused you to feel time pressured, to eat on the run, and to overeat foods that drain your energy and health. So in addition to helping you to gain control over food, eat healthier, and lose weight, I hope they will help you to feel less stressed and more energetic, and experience more pleasure at mealtimes. This chapter allows you to move from one pattern to another in any order you see fit. This flexibility empowers my patients to be more invested in their weight loss. I hope it will do the same for you.

Unguided Grazer

Weight Busters
Create a Supporting Structure

If someone asked me to identify the most important strategy for the unguided grazer, my answer would be straightforward: You need to develop a structure for eating and choosing your food. With other things in life, you probably recognize the value and benefits of maintaining structure, such as giving employees a structured workplace routine or providing children with a structured school environment. Structure can anchor your days and put some predictability into your routine. The exact same principle applies to your eating habits.

> ➢ *Nibble on This* ➢
> Give structure to your eating and you'll begin to reconfigure your figure.

The first step is to make a commitment each day to eat 3 meals without fail—morning (breakfast), afternoon (lunch), and evening (dinner). If you don't typically eat in the morning, just the thought of it may make you feel a little uneasy or even sick to your stomach (some call it morning anorexia)—which is how some of my patients react when I first make this suggestion. If that's you, start off with something small, like multigrain toast, instant oatmeal, a high-fiber bagel, or a nutrition bar such as Luna or Slim-Fast. Over time, you will obtain an appetite and move into a more nutritious breakfast. For other meals, think about what you need to do to establish a routine, such as bringing lunch from home or eating healthier meals on the road. You may find that a midmorning or late-afternoon snack wards off excessive hunger later in the day. Once you start eating regularly, you will be surprised at the energy boost this simple ritual gives you.

Just Eat—and Enjoy

Making a conscious effort to just eat when you're eating is next. This may be novel for grazers, who are more used to accompanying their meals with competing activities such as surfing the Net, driving their cars, riding in an elevator, or talking on the phone. These activities can easily distract grazers from really enjoying their food and even from eating healthier as they rush through their meals. In our sped-up world, one of the great ironies is that we talk about loving food but we don't take the time truly to experience it. It's ironic because many people don't even taste or see the food they are consuming.

So I encourage you to slow down your eating—and enjoy. One strategy is key: Put down your fork and knife at regular intervals and chew all of your food. As you eat more slowly and tune in to your appetite, you can gauge your portions around your feelings of hunger and fullness.

> ⮞ *Nibble on This* ⮜
> It takes about 20 minutes for the mind and body to register fullness.

Don't be surprised if you need much less food to feel full. My patients are often surprised at how even in the midst of a busy workday there are small things they can do to increase their mealtime enjoyment. For one patient, the simple act of closing his office door and letting voice mail pick up his messages during lunchtime helped him to focus on nourishing and energizing both his mind and body. For another, setting her alarm just 15 minutes earlier enabled her to start her day on the right health track with breakfast. Still another stopped eating behind the wheel so he could enjoy his meal without worrying about traffic. Think about the easy changes you can make that will bring pleasurable eating (and more control) back into your routine.

Connect Your Hunger and Fullness Cues

Once you are eating with fewer distractions, you can start to pay attention to something you've probably been ignoring for a long time—your hunger and fullness cues. Disconnected from their natural biological clocks, grazers either never feel hunger—since they typically don't pay attention to these vital cues—or they don't eat for hours on end until they are famished, at which time they eat whatever can be purchased, prepared, or heated up the quickest. Others eat continuously because they never feel full. As you learn to sense what and when to eat, you'll be well on your way to regaining control of your weight.

If you're in the first camp and don't know what hunger feels like, it's time to do a test. After eating breakfast, inventory yourself every hour or so for this internal signal. The actual sensation of hunger varies from localized growling, rumbling, gnawing, or emptiness of the stomach to headache, fatigue, or jitteriness. Don't eat until you begin to feel these sensations and note the time since breakfast. Just as the sensation of hunger varies among people, so does the time interval needed between meals. It is important that you detect what your body needs and when. And if you notice that you're less hungry after eating some protein at lunch (such as peanut butter on a bagel) or a fiber-filled dinner (such as extra vegetables and lentil soup), then you can use this information to your advantage when planning your meals. The better you are at detecting and controlling your hunger cues, the more in control you will be.

If you don't eat until you are famished, then you are likely ignoring early hunger signs. The solution here is to start eating on a predetermined schedule, not allowing more than about 4 hours between meals or snacks. By warding off feelings of starvation, you will be more in control and have the focus and time to select healthier foods.

Another equally important sensation for grazers to detect is fullness—the biological signal that tells you to stop eating. If you say you don't get full, I recommend stopping every 5 minutes to see how you feel so that you take inventory of your senses as you eat.

> ⇝ *Nibble on This* ⇜
> Taking a midmeal break can break your pattern of never feeling full.

Fill up on Fiber and Water

Drink more water—about 64 ounces or 8 glasses each day is the general rule. You can carry a plastic bottle with you throughout the day so that you can hydrate your body consistently and give it the essential nutrient it needs for optimal functioning. Sports nutritionists have found that hunger is often the first sign of dehydration. If you feel hungry between meals, try drinking an 8-ounce glass of water and then waiting a few moments. Chances are you will feel content. It's also a good practice to drink a glass of water before each meal. By first filling your stomach with fluid, you can take the edge off a craving or decrease feelings of intense hunger.

If you don't believe that eating fiber-filled foods will ward off grazing throughout the day, try this simple test. Eat a high-fiber cereal for breakfast such as Fiber One or Shredded Wheat N'Bran. If you're not used to the taste, sprinkle sugar substitute on top, and feel free to mix with one of your old favorites. Top with blueberries (which of course adds even more fiber) and some skim milk, then pay attention to your sense of hunger or fullness.

If you find that you're ravenous at the same time each afternoon, a higher-fiber lunch is in order. Turn a simple lunch salad into a satisfying meal by topping it with beans or accompanying it with a cup of bean soup. And if you choose to include snacks, select one that is short on calories (200 calories or fewer) and long on fiber, such as a fresh apple or pear, low-fat yogurt with a high-fiber cereal sprinkled on top, or even a fiber-rich cookie.

If eating just one higher-fiber meal a day can decrease hunger, imagine how eating more fiber consistently throughout the day can make you feel. I recommend that you shoot for 25 to 38 grams of fiber intake per day. Yes, you may have more gas (at least initially), but if you progress slowly with this strategy and increase water intake along with the fiber, your body will adapt. The tables below give you some fiber food facts so you can make better choices.

Fiber Finder: Cereals

Cereal	Calories/Serving Size	Fiber Grams
Fiber One (General Mills)	60 (½ cup)	14
All Bran (Kellogg's)	80 (½ cup)	10
Go Lean (Kashi)	120 (¾ cup)	10
Good Friends Cinna-Raisin Crunch (Kashi)	150 (1 cup)	10
Shredded Wheat N' Bran (Post)	200 (1¼ cups)	8
Shredded Wheat Spoon Size (Post)	170 (1 cup)	6
Wheat Chex (General Mills)	180 (1 cup)	5
Complete Wheat Bran Flakes (Kellogg's)	90 (¾ cup)	5
Bran Flakes (Post)	100 (¾ cup)	5
Puffins (Barbara's Bakery)	90 (¾ cup)	5
Multigrain Shredded Spoonfuls (Barbara's Bakery)	120 (¾ cup)	4
Multi Grain Cheerios* (General Mills)	110 (1 cup)	3
Whole Grain Total* (General Mills)	110 (¾ cup)	3
Grape Nut Flakes* (Post)	110 (¾ cups)	3
Whole Grain Wheaties* (General Mills)	110 (1 cup)	3

Note: High-fiber cereals contain more than 5 grams fiber; good source of fiber cereals contain 2.5–5 grams.
Try mixing cereals to enhance flavor.
*Has hydrogenated oils (trans fats).

Fiber Finder: Beans, Grain, and Soy Products

Food Category & Item	Calories/Serving Size	Fiber grams
Canned Beans *(rinse to reduce sodium and gas production)*		
Great northern beans	110 (½ cup)	7
Garbanzo beans	80 (½ cup)	7
Kidney beans	110 (½ cup)	6
Black beans	100 (½ cup)	5
Vegetarian Baked Beans (Heinz)	140 (½ cup)	5
Bean Soups		
Microwave Black Bean (Safeway Select)	170 (1 container)	14
Microwave Black Bean (Nile)	170 (1 container)	12
Hearty Black Bean (Progresso)	170 (1 cup)	10
Lentil (Progresso)	140 (1 cup)	7
Green Split Pea (Progresso)	170 (1 cup)	5
Microwave Tex-Mex Rice & Beans (Safeway Select)	200 (1 container)	5
Grains		
Whole Wheat Spaghetti (Hodgson Mill)	190 (2 ounces dry; 1 cup cooked)	6
Prince Healthy Harvest Whole Wheat Blend Pasta (thin spaghetti)	210 (2 ounces dry; 1 cup cooked)	3
Barley	170 (¼ cup dry)	5
Oats	150 (½ cup dry)	4
Quinoa	160 (¼ cup dry)	3
Oatmeal, instant	130 (1 packet)	3
Brown rice	170 (¼ cup)	2
Polenta	80 (4 ounce)	2
Wheat Germ, Original Toasted (Kretschmer)	50 (2 tablespoons)	2
Breads		
Brainy Bagel (Natural Ovens)†	170 (1 bagel)	6
Multigrain Stay Trim Bread (Natural Ovens)†	60 (1 slice)	5
Hunger Filler Whole Grain Bread (Natural Ovens)†	60 (1 slice)	5

Fiber Finder: Beans, Grains, and Soy Products

Food Category & Item	Calories/Serving Size	Fiber grams
Breads		
Whole wheat pita	140 (1 4-inch size)	4
Hearty 100% Whole Grain (Healthy Choice)	80 (1 slice)	3
100% Whole Wheat* (Brownberry)	90 (1 slice)	3
English muffin, honey wheat (Thomas')	130 (1 muffin)	2
Crackers		
Natural Ry-Krisp	60 (2 crackers)	4
Seasoned Ry-Krisp*	60 (2 crackers)	3
RyVita Whole Grain Crispbread	70 (2 slices)	3
Soy/Veggie Products		
Chicken-Style Seitan (White Wave)	130 (1 piece)	10
Edamame (boiled soybeans)	90 (½ cup)	8
Boca Burgers*	110 (1 burger)	4
Boca Crumbles (great substitute for ground beef)	70 (½ cup)	2
Soy milk (Sunsoy)	80 (1 cup)	less than 1

*Has hydrogenated oils (trans fats).
†Call 1-800-558-3535 to order Natural Ovens products or for more information.

Success Boosters

Now that your eating no longer has to fluctuate with varying work and social schedules, you're feeling more energetic and much more in control. And planning ahead has probably helped you to feel less stressed and to choose more nourishing foods. More predictability in your routine and food choices means more predictability in your weight loss. Check your progress with these questions:

	Yes	No
■ Am I eating regular meals and snacks most days?	____	____
■ Am I eating more meals without multitasking?	____	____
■ Am I enjoying my meals more?	____	____

- Am I eating more often in response to hunger?   ____   ____
- Am I identifying my fullness and stopping signals?   ____   ____
- Am I eating more fiber-filled foods?   ____   ____
- Am I drinking more water?   ____   ____

Nighttime Nibbler

Weight Busters
Redistribute Your Calories

> ➣ *Nibble on This* ➢
>
> The solution to your night eating problems begins with your daytime eating habits.

Though seemingly counterintuitive, the winning strategy for night eating is to change the way you eat during the day. If you fill up at night only, your body can't burn those calories effectively and they end up getting stored as sugar and fat.

To break the habit, plan to eat lunch and a midafternoon snack each day. Lunch doesn't have to be heavy, a sandwich or yogurt or soup is fine. The late-afternoon snack can be an apple and reduced fat peanut butter or low-fat string cheese and crackers. Carbohydrate and protein combination snacks like these are quite satisfying.

These changes alone result in better control, less night eating, and a change in appetite. You'll find that you begin feeling hungrier in the morning. That's the time to add a morning meal to your routine.

Calorieproof Your Home

As long as you have your favorite nighttime munchies (ice cream, chips, cookies, candy bars, and other baked goods) around the house, breaking your night eating habit will be hard. The solution is quite simple: Get rid of them! Just as I tell smokers who are trying to stop to throw out all of their cigarettes, remove all ashtrays, and clean their house and car to freshen the air, I tell nibblers to remove the old snacks and replace them with healthier ones. Keep a bowl of fresh fruit on the counter. If others in the household demand to have their snacks around, ask them to hide them out of sight to make it easier for you. Better yet, ask family members to try healthier snacks. You and your family can still enjoy your favorite foods within moderation, but it will be easier for all of you if they're not kept around the house.

Janyce caught on to the idea of calorieproofing her house when she remembered using a similar tactic of "out of sight, out of mind" for her five-year-old son who kept getting into mischief with her husband's carpenter tools. The most sensible solution was to "dangerproof" the house by hiding the tools. She went through her kitchen with a similar mind-set of looking for dangerous foods, that is, foods she (and her husband) got into trouble with during their evening forays. Out went the cookies, candy bars, chips, and her most favorite snack, Dove Bars. She replaced these temptations with fiber-rich cookies, baked chips, fat-free fudgsicles, frozen, low-fat yogurt, frozen mango slices, and fresh melons when in season—all lower in calories than her usual fare. By shifting to healthier snack choices, she shaved hundreds of calories a day from her diet and, along with the other nibbler strategies, she eventually cured her long-term nocturnal habit.

Plan One Nightly Snack That Satisfies

Although it is okay to treat yourself to an after-dinner snack, it needs to be planned and it needs to be just one. Decide on one snack for the night that is healthier than you would usually eat and something you would enjoy. Examples are sweet cherries, low-calorie ice cream sandwich, fat-free pudding, or popcorn. Eat slowly and enjoy. If you are still hungry, I suggest filling up on a glass of water, a sugar-free beverage like Crystal Light, or herbal tea. See the following list of other satisfying snacks.

Snack Foods

Food Category & Item	Calories*/Serving Size	Fiber grams*
Fruit Snacks		
Apple	80 (1 medium w/ skin) 70 (1 medium w/o skin)	4 (with skin) 2.5 (w/o skin)
Apricots	50 (3 medium)	2.5
Banana	53 (½ medium)	1.5
Blackberries	40 (½ cup)	4
Blueberries	40 (½ cup)	2
Cantaloupe	30 (½ cup)	1
Cherries	50 (10 cherries)	2
Grapefruit	40 (½ medium)	1.5
Grapes	60 (1 cup)1	
Guava	50 (1 medium)	5
Honeydew melon	60 (1 cup)1	
Kiwi	50 (1 medium)	3
Mango	70 (½ medium)	2
Nectarine	70 (1 medium)	2
Orange	60 (1 medium)	3
Papaya	30 (¼ medium)	1.5
Peach	40 (1 medium)	2
Pear	100 (1 medium)	4
Pineapple	40 (½ cup)	1
Plum	40 (1 medium)	1
Raspberries	30 (½ cup)	4
Strawberries	25 (½ cup)	2
Tangerine	40 (1 medium)	2
Watermelon	25 (½ cup)	less than 1
Veggie Snacks		
Broccoli	12 (½ cup)	1.5
Carrots	30 (1 medium)	2
Cauliflower	15 (½ cup)	1.5
Celery	10 (1 stalk)	less than 1
Cucumbers	10 (½ cup slices)	less than 1

Snack Foods *(cont.)*

Hearts of palm	10 (1 heart)	less than 1
Mushrooms	10 (½ cup)	less than 1
Peppers, sweet	15 (½ cup)	less than 1
Radishes	10 (10 radishes)	less than 1
Spinach	6 (½ cup)	less than 1
Tomato	30 (1 tomato)	1.5
Dairy Snacks		
Light string cheese	50 (1 piece)	0
Yoplait Light Nonfat Yogurt	100 (6 ounces)	0
Carb and Protein Combos		
Light Laughing Cow cheese and Natural Ry-Krisp crackers	90 total 30 (1 cheese wedge) 60 (2 crackers)	3
Cottage cheese and fruit slices	120 total 80 (½ cup cottage cheese) 40 (1 peach)	2
Apple and reduced-fat peanut butter†	175 total 80 (1 apple) 95 (1 tablespoon peanut butter)	5
Sargento Light Swiss Cheese and Ryvita Light Rye Whole Grain Crispbread	140 total 80 (1 slice cheese) 70 (2 crackers)	3
Whole wheat pita and hummus	190 total 140 (1 pita) 50 (2 tablespoons hummus)	7
Baked Tostitos chips and Bearitos vegetarian bean dip	135 total 110 (20 chips) 25 (2 tablespoons dip)	3
Cucumbers, tomatoes, light string cheese cut up, and Kraft Fat Free Ranch Dressing	140 total 10 (½ cup cucumbers) 30 (1 tomato) 50 (1 string cheese) 50 (2 tablespoons dressing)	2
Yoplait Light Nonfat Yogurt topped with Fiber One cereal	130 total 100 (6 ounces yogurt) 30 (¼ cup cereal)	7
Other Processed Snacks		
Jell-O Fat Free Chocolate Vanilla Swirl Pudding Snacks	100 (1 snack)	less than 1

Snack Foods *(cont.)*

Natural Ovens Chip-Mate Cookies‡	90 (1 cookie)	3
Nature Valley Oats n Honey Granola Bar	90 (1 bar)	1–2
Quaker Low-Fat Granola Bars†	110 (1 bar)	1
GeniSoy Soy Crisps Roasted Garlic and Onion (www.genisoy.com)	100 (25 crisps)	2
Orville Redenbacher's Caramel Popcorn Cakes	40 (1 cake)	1–2
Pop-Secret 94% fat free butter popcorn†	55 (3 cups popped)	2
Rold Gold Pretzel Rods†	110 (3 pretzels)	1
Quaker Instant Oatmeal Maple & Brown Sugar	160 (1 packet)	3
Hershey's Tastetation candies	20 (1 candy)	0
Frozen Snacks		
Frozen Mixed Berries (strawberries, blackberries, blueberries, raspberries)	80 (¾ cup)	4
Silhouette Low Fat Ice Cream Sandwich† Chocolate Peanut Butter Cup (www.skinnycow.com)	140 (1 sandwich)	2
Welch's Fruit Juice Bars	45 (1 bar)	0
Good Humor Fat free Fudgsicle	60 (1)	less than 1
1 Keebler Waffle bowl† with ½ cup Edy's Fat Free Frozen Yogurt (black cherry vanilla swirl) and ½ cup fresh raspberries	170 (total) 50 (bowl) 90 (yogurt) 30 (fruit)	2
Diana's Bananas Banana Babies (chocolate-dipped frozen bananas)	140 (1)	3
Healthy Choice Low Fat Ice Cream†	120 (½ cup)	less than 1
Banana, dipped in water, rolled in honey crunch wheat germ, and then frozen	135 total 105 (1 medium banana) 30 (1 tablespoon wheat germ)	3
Miscellaneous		
Edamame (boiled soybeans)	90 (½ cup)	8
Pickles, dill	5 (1 spear)	less than 1

Sources: Food labels and Jean J. T. Pennington, *Bowe's & Church's Food Values of Portions Commonly Used.*

*Calorie and fiber values have been rounded off.

†Has hydrogenated oils (trans fats).

‡Call 1-800-558-3535 to order Natural Ovens products or for more information.

You may be questioning if you can limit yourself to just one after-dinner snack. Here, the key to being successful starts with having a satisfying dinner—one that is filling and nutritious. I'm not talking about overeating and feeling stuffed, but rather feeling satisfied and content. Adding fiber to your dinner in the form of fruits, vegetables, and whole-grain foods is a sure bet to ward off hunger for hours after the meal. This strategy speaks to many nighttime nibblers who are used to eating dinners that are quite low in fiber. Look back at your food diary and see if your typical dinner meal contains the following:

- 1 or more servings of fruit
- 1 or more servings of vegetables
- 1 or more servings of beans or legumes
- 1 serving of whole grains (whole-grain bread, pasta, or crackers, brown rice; barley; wild rice)

To maximize your fiber intake at dinner, add some of these foods while cutting your main course protein—chicken, beef, or fish—down to 4 ounces, the size of a deck of cards or a cassette (see Chapter 7 for recipes). Or toss canned kidney beans or chickpeas (drained and rinsed) onto your side salad or have a cup of split pea soup before your main dish. Consider eating more fruit and vegetable side dishes. Once nighttime nibblers start eating more fiber-rich dinners, they feel more satisfied and able to follow this important strategy.

Reset Your Nighttime Routine

"My habits override my brain," commented Mike. A manager of a large restaurant chain (and a classic nighttime nibbler), he spent his days rushing from one franchise office to another, checking on business and putting out fires along the way. On a typical day, he would down a large coffee mid-morning and bits of food here and there the rest of the day. By the time he arrived home at 7 P.M., he was starved and couldn't eat fast enough. A large dinner spilled over into evening snacking until 11 P.M., when he crashed into bed. My treatment started with adding a scheduled lunch and a late-afternoon snack, which decreased feelings of intense hunger at dinnertime. Though his wife replaced some high-calorie snack foods with healthier alternatives, cookies and ice cream remained at home for the kids' after-school treats. And Mike still couldn't resist them.

More than needing information, Mike needed to analyze and ultimately reset—called behavior modification by professionals—his nighttime routine. If you have rituals at night that make it hard to change your eating habits, you too will need to take a closer look at your routine. What you have developed, quite naturally, is a pairing of several behaviors: watching television in a favorite comfort chair AND eating caramel corn; sitting on the couch reading the newspaper AND munching on chips, or lying in bed to watch the evening news AND snacking on a bowl of ice cream.

You need to untangle the associations: Change chairs or even rooms for watching television; decide that the bedroom's off-limits for eating; brush your teeth after your one nightly snack to reinforce that eating is over for the night. In Mike's case, he discovered that his nightly routine of putting his feet up, listening to music, reading the newspaper, AND eating cookies and ice cream were all linked to unwinding after very stressful days. I showed him that he could unwind without the food, but he needed to change his ritual. So instead of plopping down on the same chair each night, he went to a different room where he never ate. The change in routine disconnected the eating, and he found it easier now for his "brain to override his habits."

Success Boosters

Now that you're retiring to bed less full and waking up less full, you're feeling more energetic throughout the day and much more in control of your night eating. Some of my patients have even seen their sex lives improve— all good signs as your body is positively adjusting to your new lifestyle. Check your progress with these questions:

	Yes	No
■ Am I eating more during the day?	____	____
■ Am I eating more fiber-filled foods at dinner?	____	____
■ Am I eating less after dinner?	____	____
■ Am I enjoying one planned healthy snack per night?	____	____
■ Have I changed my nighttime routine?	____	____

Convenient Consumer

Weight Busters
Downsize, Don't Supersize

With supersize meals easily containing more than half your daily requirement for both calories and heart-clogging fat, my first tactic here involves doing the numbers game to show you just how downsizing works (see table below). For example, if you substitute your usual Burger King fare of a double whopper with cheese, king fries, and medium cola (1,840 calories) with a Jr. whopper (hold the mayo), child onion rings, and medium diet cola, you cut your calories by 1,300. If you downsized similarly during each weekly visit to Burger King for a year, you'd lose about 19 pounds (if your activity level was also increased to combat your decreasing metabolism as your weight dropped). The point is that downsizing really works to shed the pounds. And the same illustration could be done with every fast-food chain in America, most of which have their nutritional information available in pamphlets (ask for one if you don't see them) or on wall posters. Some even have interactive Web sites.

Some patients are initially concerned about being able to enjoy these downsized meals. I remind them that they're not going from a Big Mac to a roasted McTofu sandwich. Instead, you can downsize to the plain hamburger or, better yet, transition to a chicken McGrill sandwich (and replace the mayo with mustard). By making these simple substitutions, you can save yourself hundreds of calories, be on your way to losing weight, and still enjoy your customary flavors and foods.

Fast Foods Meal Comparisons

Fast-Food Restaurant	Usual Meal	Downsized Meal	Further Downsized Meal	Calorie Savings
McDonald's www.mcdonalds.com	Big Extra with cheese, super fry, super cola (1,850 calories)	Quarter pounder (no cheese), small fry, medium diet cola (750 calories)	Chicken McGrill (without mayo), chicken caesar salad with fat-free herb vinaigrette, water (470 calories)	1,100–1,380
Burger King www.burgerking.com	Double whopper with cheese, king fries, medium cola (1,840 calories)	Jr. whopper (without mayo), child onion ring, medium diet cola (540 calories)	BK broiler (without mayo), garden salad with light Italian dressing, water (500 calories)	1,300–1,340

Taco Bell www.tacobell.com	Nachos bell grande and beef Santa Fe chalupa, large cola (1,490 calories)	Soft chicken taco supreme and bean burrito, medium diet cola (610 calories)	Bean burrito or soft chicken taco and pinto beans, water (370 calories)	880–1,120
Kentucky Fried Chicken www.kentuckyfried chicken.com	Twister, wedges, large cola (1,134 calories)	Original sandwich, wedges, small diet cola (604 calories)	Tender roast sandwich, potatoes and gravy, water (390 calories)	530–744

Source: Dawn Jackson, RD, Wellness Institute, Northwestern Memorial Hospital.

So how can you downsize most painlessly? The best way is to plan ahead and know what you are going to order before you walk inside or drive through the pickup lane. If you wait until you're in the fast-food restaurant and looking up at the menu choices, it's too late—habit will likely win over. So rehearse it in your mind and tell yourself your plan. If, however, you are continuously drawn to order the same high-calorie meal that got you into larger-size clothes in the first place, then don't go to that restaurant, at least not for a while.

Downsizing convenient foods at home is another winning strategy. If you're purchasing frozen entrées, downsize the calorie level by comparing food labels. Healthy Choice, Lean Cuisine, and Weight Watchers Smart Ones are good choices, although the sodium level is a bit high in some products. And remember that downsizing *never* means going hungry. It means reducing your intake of foods with unhealthy and concentrated calories and filling up on more nutritious (preferably fiber-filled), lower-calorie ones—like fruits and vegetables. If your Lean Cuisine dinner doesn't fill you up, enjoy a large side spinach salad topped with walnuts. If you're often on the run, you can do well by grabbing an already downsized liquid meal replacement drink or bar (like Slim-Fast or Sweet Success) for a 220-calorie or less quick breakfast or lunch.

As for downsizing your snack foods, it's best to buy individually wrapped single servings and limit yourself to just one. Tasty examples include a 60-calorie Good Humor Fat Free Fudgsicle or a 45-calorie Welch's fruit juice bar. As the following table shows, reading the label, especially the calories per serving *and* the serving sizes, will give you the complete calorie story. As you can see, choosing Michael's Reduced Fat Chips means you can eat double the number of Sun Chips—without doubling the calories!

Calories per Serving Size Comparisons

Chips	Calories per Serving	Serving Size
Doritos Extreme Zesty Sour Cream and Cheddar	140	7 chips
Sun Chips French Onion Multigrain Snacks	140	10 chips
Doritos Nacho Cheesier	140	11 chips
Michael Season's Lightly Salted Potato Chips, Reduced Fat	140	20 chips

Divide and Conquer

Divide and conquer is a restaurant strategy my patient Edith developed and regularly uses to control her weight. Edith's position as an art collector for a local museum demanded that she conduct business over lunch and dinner in upscale restaurants. She couldn't pass on meals since she was the host and wanted to make a good impression. She also wanted to make her clients feel comfortable ordering anything they wished as well. So she began ordering a half portion when available, sharing an entrée with someone else, or taking half of it home. Many restaurants accommodate patrons by splitting the meal in the kitchen or bringing an empty plate to the table for splitting. Another approach is to order from the appetizer side of the menu (staying away, of course, from fried options). If you're still hungry, order soup, a side of vegetables, or a salad.

> ➣ *Nibble on This* ➢
>
> When ordering in a restaurant, assume that the usual portion sizes are large enough to feed at least a twosome.

Find Hidden Calories

Though convenient consumption may seem synonymous with high fat and high calories, there are ways you can eat both conveniently and nutritiously. Begin by striking "fried" from your vocabulary and replace it with "baked," "broiled," "grilled," "roasted," or "boiled." *Baked* potato chips, *broiled* fish, *grilled* chicken, *roasted* vegetables, *boiled* egg—you get the idea. Frying takes perfectly healthy foods and transforms them into unhealthy, higher-calorie foods. The major difficulty isn't finding healthier alternatives—the food industry actually makes them readily available. The difficulty lies in learning to change your taste buds, especially if you've enjoyed fried foods your whole life. The solution is to experiment with an assortment of spices and condiments, such as a grilled chicken breast jazzed up with fresh rosemary or tarragon, or marinated in teriyaki or a spicy barbecue sauce. It takes a few weeks to adapt to a new taste, so don't give up.

> ⇒ *Nibble on This* ⇐
>
> When you practice avoiding hidden calories, you often uncover hidden flavors you enjoy.

Other sources of hidden calories include cream sauces, salad dressings, mayo, butter, and margarine. As a rule, either order these on the side or, better, substitute with non- or low-calorie alternatives like mustard and low-fat dressings. Liquid calories in the form of colas, sodas, fruit juices, and wine and other alcoholic beverages can also quickly add up. And many foods, such as cakes, pastries, croissants, and cheeses, truly contain hidden calories since fat is in the products and can't be removed. Either eat them in moderation or, once again, substitute, such as choosing a multigrain bread over a croissant. See the table below for more menu maneuvers.

Menu Maneuvers

Restaurant	Choose Smart	Avoid Food Traps	Special Requests
Fast Food	■ Side salads ■ Chili or bean soups ■ Low-fat milk ■ Bean burritos ■ Whole-grain bagel with hummus ■ Lean turkey or roast beef sandwich ■ Baked potato and salsa ■ Grilled instead of fried chicken sandwich ■ Small hamburger	■ Mayonnaise, sauce, or creamy salad dressing ■ Fried chicken or fish ■ French fries ■ Soft drinks ■ Fatty meats ■ Breakfast sandwiches	■ Hold the mayo ■ Extra lettuce, tomatoes, pickles, onions ■ Leanest meat ■ No cheese on sandwich ■ Sauce on side ■ Vinaigrette instead of creamy dressing

Menu Maneuvers *(cont.)*

Restaurant	Choose Smart	Avoid Food Traps	Special Requests
American	■ Noncream soup ■ Salads ■ Lean meats ■ Grain dishes	■ Large main course portion size ■ Foods fried or sautéed ■ Cream sauce and dressings	■ Take home half of main course or share ■ Choose appetizer or lunch-size item for dinner ■ Whole-grain rolls or bread ■ Moderate olive oil instead of butter ■ Sauce or dressing on side ■ Light on the oil ■ Vegetable of the day or extra vegetable at dinner
Italian	■ Bean and pasta soup ■ Whole-grain pasta with veggies and oil or wine-based sauce ■ Pasta marinara (no meat) ■ Salad ■ Veggies ■ Thin-crust pizza with a little cheese and extra vegetables	■ Alfredo or other cream-based sauce ■ Cheese-based grain dishes ■ Double-cheese pizza ■ Garlic bread ■ Large portions with rich sauces ■ Fried eggplant	■ Hold the cheese or light on the cheese ■ Add veggies to pizza ■ Plain bread with olive oil ■ Light on sauce or oil and take half home or share ■ Glass, not bottle, of wine
Asian (Thai, Chinese, etc.)	■ Rice and noodle dishes with lots of vegetables ■ Brown rice dishes when available ■ Tofu (bean curd) dishes ■ Fish and seafood ■ Broth-based soups	■ Deep-fried appetizers or dishes ■ Crispy noodles ■ Sweet and sour dishes ■ Curry dishes made with coconut milk ■ Mee krob (fried crispy noodles)	■ Cook food light on oil ■ Brown rice instead of white ■ Chopsticks help you to eat slower and more mindfully
Japanese	■ Broth-based soup ■ Sushi ■ California or vegetable rolls ■ Fish and seafood ■ Edamame ■ Other rice dishes	■ Deep-fried dishes such as tempura	■ Take home half of fish entrée or share
Indian	■ Grain dishes with vegetables, lentils, beans ■ Salads with yogurt ■ Roasted tandoori-style meats	■ Deep-fried breads and appetizers ■ Ghee (clarified butter) used in cooking	■ Leaner meats ■ Light on butter or oils ■ Make without cream

Restaurant	Choose Smart	Avoid Food Traps	Special Requests
Middle Eastern/Greek	▪ Bean or lentil soups ▪ Hummus and pita ▪ Fish ▪ Rice and couscous dishes ▪ Shish kebab with chicken or lean beef	▪ Fried cheese	▪ Light on oil ▪ Whole-grain pita
Mexican	▪ Vegetarian dishes ▪ Bean dishes ▪ Rice dishes ▪ Salads ▪ Bean soup ▪ Gazpacho ▪ Chili ▪ Soft tacos ▪ Fajitas	▪ Deep-fried tortillas or chips ▪ Chimichanga	▪ Soft tortillas with the salsa ▪ Hold the cheese ▪ Substitute lite sour cream ▪ Salsa instead of guacamole ▪ Limit margaritas, sangria

I encourage you to plan your attack before you enter the restaurant. You'll arrive prepared not to order anything "as is" off the menu since many menus feature large portions with hidden fats. Try new foods (and new restaurants) when eating out. Even though ethnic restaurants have gotten a bad rap for dieters, their choices are often rich in vegetables and whole grains and lower in animal fat. Pay attention to the types of restaurants in which you're able to eat healthier portions and the ones that more typically set you up to overeat. Also, if you overeat in a restaurant, do not to feel guilty or beat yourself up about it. Instead, think about how you can eat healthier next time.

> ⮞ *Nibble on This* ⮜
> When ordering off a menu, order it your way—not their way.

When taking an Asian cooking class, Nancy was surprised at how much oil the teacher used before adding *each* vegetable ingredient to the wok. The teacher said that the extra oil speeds up the cooking time and is a technique commonly used in restaurants. Whenever I eat Asian food, I now ask that the food be cooked with a light amount of oil. Try this simple request. You probably won't even taste the difference. I didn't.

Cooking, Anyone?

Trying to be a convenient chef—at least once in a while—may seem like an oxymoron to a convenient consumer. But it's a strategy I suggest if you want to shed more pounds. Some of my patients are ashamed to admit that they haven't prepared a home-cooked meal for months. Tracy was one of them, with a diet that consisted of 100 percent preprepared foods: morning coffee and doughnut, fast-food submarine sandwich lunch, and takeout Chinese, Thai, or pizza for dinner. The first three strategies—downsize, divide and conquer, and find hidden calories—helped Tracy to lose 35 pounds over 4 months, but instead of being content and stopping there, she discovered the joys of cooking. She went from assembling simple (and still convenient) meals like a frozen medley of chicken, vegetables, and pasta mixed with an extra bag of frozen vegetables to learning how to grill chicken, roast vegetables, and create colorful salads. Tracy was never one to eat a piece of fruit, but she loved cut-up fruit salads, which she quickly became an expert at preparing. Before long, she became the envy of her other convenient consumer friends as she sponsored cooking parties and had loads of fun to boot. Gaining better control through her home-prepared meals allowed Tracy to lose even more weight.

I encourage convenient consumers to get cooking inspiration from their favorite healthy restaurant meals. One patient noticed that capers and grilled chicken turned a simple Greek salad into a delicious and healthy entrée salad, which was easy to copy at home. Another patient used ready-made pizza crusts and cooked chicken strips to copy an Asian style specialty pizza that she loved. Another had a home cooking party through the Pampered Chef, where they do cooking demonstrations and sell professional quality kitchen tools. And still another learned a lot just by watching television cooking shows and reading healthy cooking magazines (trying one new recipe each month). To help you build confidence in the kitchen, try some of our recipe ideas in Chapter 7 and you may surprise yourself—and your family—with your newfound culinary skills.

> ⮞ *Nibble on This* ⮜
>
> Imitation is the best form of flattery. While sampling healthier foods in restaurants, ask about the ingredients and preparation of the dishes you like—and try to copy them at home.

Success Boosters

Now that supersize portions of fast food, movie food, or even drinks at convenience stores don't tempt you the way they used to, you're feeling much more in control of your eating. Instead of thinking about them as great deals where you can get the most for your money, you realize they're really "poor health deals" that rob you of your energy and undermine your personal best. Check your progress with these questions:

	Yes	No
■ Am I downsizing, not supersizing?	___	___
■ Am I enjoying my downsized meals?	___	___
■ Am I planning ahead before I eat out?	___	___
■ Am I downsizing at home also?	___	___
■ Am I scrutinizing the calories per serving size on food labels?	___	___
■ Have I found snack foods that are convenient, healthy, and satisfying?	___	___
■ Am I dividing and conquering when eating out?	___	___
■ Am I avoiding fried foods, cream sauces, creamy salad dressings, mayo, butter, and margarine?	___	___
■ Am I making special (and healthier) requests in restaurants?	___	___
■ Have I tried cooking simple dishes?	___	___

Fruitless Feaster

Weight Busters
Get Fresh

First, start *adding* what is missing from your diet. You may wonder how this strategy will help you to shed pounds. It's really quite simple. The high water content of fruits and vegetables fills you up—so you're not hungry all the time. And ounce for ounce, fruits and vegetables are lower in calories than almost any other food. My most successful patients are those who adopt the mind-set that if they want to lose weight, then fruits and vegetables need to be a regular part of their daily diet. Keep trying new kinds, prepared in new ways—until you find what you most enjoy.

To consume at least 5 servings a day, add a fruit and/or vegetable to every meal, and replace most snacks with the same. It's really quite easy to do.

➣ *Nibble on This* ➢

Think of your stomach as a bucket—only so big and able to handle a finite amount of food, at least comfortably. If you first fill up on lower-calorie fruits and vegetables, you will naturally displace other higher-calorie foods from your diet.

At breakfast:

- Add blueberries, strawberries, or bananas to cereal or buckwheat pancakes.
- Add mushrooms, onions, spinach, green peppers, or salsa to omelets.
- Eat orange or melon slices with whole-grain waffles.
- Eat sliced tomatoes and cucumber on your bagel.

At lunch and dinner:

- Pack cherry tomatoes, baby carrots, cucumber slices, jicama, and orange or apple slices in your bag lunches, or add fresh berries to your yogurt.

- Add lettuce, baby spinach, arugula, tomatoes, or onions to sandwiches.
- Choose a vegetable or fresh fruit in place of french fries in restaurants.
- Add side salads to your fast-food meals.
- Add sliced apples or oranges as a side dish to any meal. Serve convenient, ready-to-eat cut up melon or pineapple with dinner.
- Learn to roast or grill vegetables.
- Grill pineapple slices alongside fish or chicken.
- Serve salads regularly as a side or main dish.

I also encourage you to notice those times when you really enjoy eating fruits and vegetables, by asking the following questions:

- Do you eat more fruits and vegetables when they're standing alone (that is, not next to other food choices)? If so, place apples or ripening pears, nectarines, peaches, mangoes, or melons in a wire basket on the counter—with the sweets out of sight and preferably out of the house. Also make sure grapes, cut-up pineapple, carrots, or celery are clean and visible in your refrigerator—and not next to the cheesecake.
- Do you eat more fruits and vegetables when you don't have to do the work preparing them? If so, choose the many ready-to-eat ones—if you are willing to pay their higher prices. Otherwise, try prepping as much produce as possible on the weekends when you have more time. Quickly wash and dry fruits and vegetables. Chop lettuce, celery, carrots, peppers, and other produce that will keep fresh in the fridge so they're ready for snacks and cooking. Engage your kids as washing and chopping helpers (you'll teach them a great lifelong health habit in the process). And put on some background music or a favorite television show.

Remember that every little bit helps. As you choose fresh over processed, you're getting the most bang for your buck by eating plant-based, nutrient-rich complex carbohydrates for the least amount of calories. My patient Elaine, a longtime fruitless feaster, came up with a creative solution for continually throwing out her uneaten and rotten fruit at home. Instead of buying fruit at the supermarket, she had fresh fruit delivered weekly to her office. She prominently placed it in a bowl in her work area. The "community fruit bowl," as her coworkers called it, was a great hit. Soon, they all chipped in to keep it stocked.

A word of caution is needed about commercial fruit juice. This is not a good way to increase your number of fruit servings. Excessive liquid calories from fruit drinks and smoothies is a major problem, particularly among kids. Since juices don't have the fiber of whole fruit, it's easy to down 8 to 12 ounces and not feel full. Depending on the juice, each ounce contains from 15 to 20 calories, which means 120 to 240 liquid calories for an 8- to 12-ounce glass. If you habitually turn to these drinks to quench your thirst, try water with a twist of lemon or other noncaloric beverages. When it comes to fruit, stick with the real thing. Many of my patients have turned to vegetable drinks such as V-8 for a morning pick-me-up. Don't allow these liquid vegetables to totally replace the real thing. Occasionally, they can be a fun and refreshing addition.

Color Your Plate

Now it's time to take a look at what you put on your plate. Is it all white (from potatoes) and yellow (from corn and bananas)? Though the first stage of change for feasters is to add fruits and vegetables, the next strategy is to add a rainbow of colorful produce that contains powerful heart disease– and cancer-fighting nutrients (phytochemicals). These compounds that give fruits and vegetables their glorious colors—red cherry tomatoes, green peppers, yellow squash, blue blueberries, dark red raspberries, and purple plums—give us energy, help to fight off disease, and keep us young. Your goal is to add as many colors to your diet as possible. If you use fresh, canned (watch sodium levels), and frozen, availability is not a problem.

> ⇒ *Nibble on This* ⇐
> Eat fruits and vegetables with intense colors to intensify healthy weight loss.

A few more words of caution on why not all fruits and vegetables are created equal. Some vegetables—potatoes, corn, and peas—are starchy, which means they are more calorie-dense than others. Don't overly rely on them when choosing fruits and veggies to eat. Also, you can take a perfectly healthy fruit or vegetable and ruin its nutritional value through frying (french fries), adding sour cream and butter (double-baked potato), cream (creamed corn), heavy syrup (canned fruits), or topping with a high-fat cheese (cheese broccoli).

Appeal to Your Senses

Fine restaurants prepare and present fruits and vegetables in visually appealing ways. Cutting, mixing, seasoning, and roasting can do wonders to enhance the flavors and tastes of fruits and vegetables while an enticing presentation stimulates the appetite. Paying more attention to these details will enhance your health and pleasure.

Kids (especially finicky ones) are often the best test cases for trying new foods. A child may refuse to snack on a large apple but savor fresh apple slices. You or your family may not think to eat whole oranges with dinner but may enjoy them on the side sliced with dried cranberries sprinkled on top. Pay attention to the little things restaurants do to boost the flavor of fruits and vegetables and copy them at home. Here are some tricks:

- *Oranges and grapefruits*. Peel oranges and pink grapefruits. Cut them into small pieces, mix them together, and store them in the refrigerator. This makes a surprisingly sweet snack or side dish.
- *Oranges and whole-berry cranberries*. Place orange slices next to slices of canned whole-berry cranberries. Makes a colorful and delicious side.
- *Berries and yogurt*. Defrost frozen berries according to package directions. In custard-type bowls, mix reduced-fat vanilla yogurt with defrosted berries. Makes a great year-round side dish or dessert.
- *Red and green apples*. Garnish your dinner plate with red and green apple slices.
- *Red and green seedless grapes*. Dust grapes with cinnamon and freeze. This makes a refreshing summertime dessert or snack.
- *Cantaloupe and blueberries*. Serve a cantaloupe wedge filled with fresh blueberries.
- *Salad greens and kiwi, strawberries, and grapes*. Top lettuce with kiwi slices, strawberries, and grapes. Drizzle with favorite light vinaigrette dressing. This makes a great summer side salad.
- *Radishes, jicama, cherry tomatoes, and yellow, green, and red pepper slices*. Serve with reduced-fat Ranch dressing.

- *Sautéed spinach.* Sauté spinach with 1 tablespoon of olive oil until wilted. Squeeze fresh lemon juice on top and serve.
- *Brussels sprouts with parmesan.* Steam brussels sprouts and lightly sprinkle with parmesan cheese. Makes a great side dish.
- *Roasted green beans.* Place washed beans on a cookie sheet greased with nonstick cooking spray. Spray green beans with cooking spray and season with garlic salt. Place in a preheated 450° oven for 40 minutes or so until beans are softened. This is a great appetizer or side dish that kids say tastes like french fries.
- *Roasted white and sweet potatoes.* Slice washed, unpeeled potatoes into wedges or french fry sticks. Place in a roasting pan greased with nonstick cooking spray. Spray potatoes with cooking spray and season with garlic powder and paprika. Place in a preheated 450° oven for an hour or so until potatoes are done. Makes a delicious dinner side dish.

Dare to Go Bare

I recommend eating a meatless dinner at least once or twice a week—just to start. I'm not talking about total vegetarianism here, but it is important to start displacing meat from your diet if you are accustomed to having meat play the lead role at every meal. My most successful patients have transformed their diet into a vegetarian delight where meat has taken second fiddle to beans, lentils, soy products, nuts, fruits, and other assorted vegetables. They've found that meatless meals allow them to eat larger portions of food—with the bonus of more fiber and fewer calories than their old meat-centered diet.

> ⪧ *Nibble on This* ⪦
> Recast fruits and vegetables to a starring role.

Many patients initially benefit from ordering meatless meals in restaurants that know how to prepare them. They frequent American, Asian, Japanese, Indian, Italian, Mexican, Middle Eastern, or even vegetarian restaurants and enjoy dishes such as vegetarian pizzas, vegetarian chili or pasta, stir-fried tofu and vegetables, edamame, vegetable maki rolls, lentil dishes, falafel, vegetable and bean fajitas, or veggie burgers. Once they taste how satisfying a dinner without meat can be, they're more motivated to prepare it at home.

Keep Boca Burgers in your freezer for a quick last-minute meal. Prepare colorful entrée salads with heart-healthy fats such as walnuts and avocados and interesting toppings such as sliced beets, garbanzo beans, chopped olives, artichokes, bean sprouts, or fresh cooked peas. Try packaged bean soups, which make a great entrée when served with a side salad and whole-grain bread. Use prepared pizza crusts to make vegetarian pizzas. See the recipes in Chapter 7 and learn how to make other meatless meals from scratch.

Success Boosters

Now that you're eating more fruits and vegetables and enjoying them, you have found that losing weight is much easier than ever before. You also notice that you don't tend to overeat these "good for you" foods the way you tended to overeat processed foods. You are feeling more energetic and more in control as your hunger level evens out. Monitor your good progress with these questions:

	Yes	No
■ Am I eating more fruits and vegetables at breakfast, lunch, dinner, and snacktime?	___	___
■ Am I eating an array of bright, colorful fruits and vegetables?	___	___
■ Am I drinking less fruit juice and eating more whole fruit?	___	___
■ Am I paying attention to times I most enjoy eating fruits and vegetables?	___	___
■ Am I adding less high-fat topping to fruits and vegetables?	___	___
■ Am I paying attention to how restaurants present healthy fruit and vegetable dishes?	___	___
■ Am I trying new fruit and vegetable presentations and combinations?	___	___
■ Am I enjoying fruits and vegetables more than I used to?	___	___

Mindless Muncher

Weight Busters
From Mindless to Conscious

The mindless muncher has difficulty accounting for all of the food and liquid calories consumed in a week—or, for that matter, even in a single day. A handful of peanuts while cooking, a taste of candy at your daughter's school, a smidgen of birthday cake at the office, a bite of your son's leftover sandwich—these unaccounted foods add literally hundreds of calories to your daily fare. For the mindless muncher, the very sight or smell of food triggers an unintentional response to eat—hungry or not. This behavior is not deliberate or a sign of weak willpower, it's simply a long-held habit of unconscious eating.

If you are a mindless muncher, you must convert your unconscious, "thoughtless" eating and drinking to conscious consumption. Awareness leads to thoughtfulness, which then ultimately leads to change. My patients quickly learn that they've been powerless to change their behaviors because they were unaware of them. As the saying goes, "If you can name them, you can tame them."

> ⋟ *Nibble on This* ⋞
>
> "In the absence of awareness, emotional reactivity and habits control your life."
>
> —Dr. Joel and Michelle Levey, *Living in Balance*

Using the food diary from Chapter 2 is the fastest way to boost awareness. By recording everything that you eat and drink over the course of a day, you become aware of every nibble, bite, and morsel of food that crosses your lips. And if you keep a diary for 3 days (or even for weeks on end, which many of my patients choose to do), some patterns to your mindless eating may soon appear. Check your diary columns for the following:

- Are there times of the day or night when mindless eating occurs more frequently?

- Are there certain types of food that lend themselves to mindless eating, such as the M&M's on your coworker's desk or the peanuts in your living room?
- Are there places where mindless eating commonly reoccurs, such as at the computer or in front of the television?
- Are there common triggers for your mindless eating, such as when you're bored at work or when you're clearing the dishes at home?
- Does your mindless eating have any relationship to hunger?

Once you can answer these questions, you're well on your way to becoming a "conscious consumer," which is the first step to taking back control. This exercise was a real eye-opener for June. She had fallen prey to the smorgasbord of free finger food that cluttered her workplace. Mindlessly, she would grab bits and pieces of snacks all day long, simply because they were there. When she began to keep a diary of her intake, not only did she become more aware of her surroundings, but she also immediately cut her robotlike eating in half. Just being more mindful got June off to a good start in changing her longtime habit. And reviewing your diary will give you a better idea of the extent and nature of your mindless eating.

Quantify Munching

This strategy helps you understand that there's munching and then there's munching, as you realize just how quickly the calories from mindless eating add up. You'll learn that counting these extra calories empowers you to make more educated choices about your diet. This strategy especially helped Mindy, who always knew she was a mindless muncher but had never really spent time trying to understand its ramifications on her weight. Just one page from her food diary showed the extra calories that added up to make her weight loss difficult.

Mindy's Food Diary

When? Time	What and How Much? Food/Beverage Portion Size Calories (optional)	Where? Home/Work/ Car/Dining Out	Why? Associated Triggers: Stimuli, Emotions, Activities	How Hungry? (0—not hungry, 4—starving)
9:00 A.M.	6 ounce yogurt ½ banana 1 dry English muffin 1 cup tea	Home	Enjoying quiet time in kitchen	3
10:30 A.M.	Cinnamon coffee cake, 1 slice	Morning program at preschool	Helping at preschool	0
Noon	Chicken salad sandwich (1 scoop) on 2 pieces wheat bread with 1 piece of lettuce 8 ounce water 1 orange	Home	Friend stopped over for lunch	2
3:30 P.M.	6 chocolate kisses	Kid's school	Third-grade celebration for oldest child; didn't want to be a party pooper and felt like I deserved a reward	1
5:30 P.M.	2 slices cheese pizza 12-ounce Diet Coke 1 cookie	Home	Dinner with children	2
8:30 P.M.	1 bag potato chips 8-ounce glass orange juice	Home	Serving late dinner to spouse; don't want him to eat alone	1

On this particular day, Mindy's mindless eating totaled 611 calories: coffee cake, 200 calories; chocolate kisses, 156; potato chips and juice, 255. If she curbed only her mindless eating, she would be well on her way to losing more than 1 pound each week! It's time now to look back at your food diary and quantify your munching, just the way Mindy did. Using food labels along with the Quick Method to Estimate Portions (page 39) is helpful here. Alternatively, a small weight scale for measuring food ounces, measuring cups and spoons, and a calorie counter are tools to use on a trial basis. And remember that looking at several days from your diary will give you the most accurate picture. For many people, mindless eating is not a problem during the week when they're busy at work and have a set routine. It's more of a problem on weekends when they're hanging out at home. If this is you,

I recommend you keep the diary for at least two weekdays and on both Saturday and Sunday.

Refresh with Healthier Alternatives

Mindless munchers typically respond well to my recommendation that they carry a water bottle with them and focus on drinking 8 glasses a day. Some enjoy the flavored waters, such as La Croix Sparkling Lemon, Lime, or Orange or Poland Spring Sparkling Lemon (read labels and stay away from the sugar-flavored, high-calorie waters). Others discover the water coolers at their offices. Still others make an investment to have bottled water delivered to their home. So the next time you want to grab for food, drink water first.

Pay attention to how your hunger level in your food diary relates to your eating. Notice that Mindy's hunger level was always low (0 or 1) during her mindless eating episodes. The next time you want to munch, rate your hunger level first. If it's a 0 or 1, drink a glass of water or do something else (practice deep breathing, take a walk, call a friend, read a magazine). If you're still hungry after a few minutes, then go ahead and eat.

> ➤ *Nibble on This* ⬅
> Hunger is often a symptom of needing water, not food.

Other snacks that can satisfy your hunger are sweet cherry tomatoes dipped in light Ranch dressing, baked chips and vegetarian bean dip, or whole wheat pita and hummus dip. If you think about the three environments (home, work, or social) where your mindless eating occurs, you want to make sure that these "better-for-you" foods are available in all settings. At home, that may mean adding some of these foods to your weekly shopping list. If you can't resist munching on salty potato chips, keep microwave popcorn or rice cakes in your cupboards. At work, that may mean keeping low-fat granola bars or cherry-covered chocolate Luna bars in your desk drawer so when a vendor brings doughnuts, you have a healthier (and still sweet) option available. And for social activities, you might choose to bring a healthy appetizer to the party or bring your own popcorn to the movies. Those patients who indulge their cravings with healthy, tasty, planned alternatives sustain more dramatic weight loss than those who simply deprive themselves of any food and ignore their cravings.

> ### ⮞ *Nibble on This* ⮜
>
> A little creative thinking goes a long way to feed your healthy eating habit. Enjoy a lower-calorie but still yummy version of kettle corn (or sweetened popcorn) by sprinkling sugar substitute onto microwave popcorn (saturated fat free).

Tame Your Triggers

The first three strategies have enabled you to be more mindful of your eating habits and to lessen its negative effects on your weight. Now it's time to take full control by stopping (or significantly diminishing) the mindless eating altogether. This can be accomplished by looking a little deeper at the triggers from your diary that precede your eating:

- snacking stimuli such as the presence of food at home, work, the movies, or gas stations
- specific activities such as preparing meals at home, attending office meetings, filling your car up with gas
- emotions such as fatigue, stress, anxiety, loneliness, boredom

The following tables show Sam's and Mindy's mindless eating records. You may notice that for a mindless muncher, there are not any serious emotional triggers except for maybe some boredom here or there, which is in sharp contrast to the emotional eater, who uses food to cope with stress, anxiety, depression, and loneliness. That's because the eating of the typical mindless muncher really is mindless!

Sam's Mindless Eating Record

Place	Related Activities	Food	Related Emotions	Strategies for Extinguishing Mindless Eating
Office	Semiweekly staff meeting	Doughnuts, coffee cake	Nothing unusual	■ Make sure to eat breakfast ■ Take water bottle to meeting and don't take plate or napkin ■ Keep healthy snacks in office
Office	Passing coworker's desk	Gummy bears, jelly beans	Nothing unusual	■ Set rules for self not to eat while standing or walking ■ Keep individually wrapped 20-calorie Tastetation candies in desk drawer for a quick low-calorie, sweet chocolate fix
On the road	Filling up car with gas	Candy bar, chips	Nothing unusual	■ Pay at the pump ■ Take water bottle in car ■ Keep healthy snacks in car

Mindy's Mindless Eating Record

Place	Related Activities	Food	Related Emotions	Strategies for Extinguishing Mindless Eating
Child's school	School meeting	Coffee cake, chocolate kisses	Nothing unusual	■ Bring water bottle to school ■ Stay away from food and instead focus on activities
Home	Serving late dinner to spouse	Potato chips, juice	Nothing unusual	■ Drink a glass of water ■ Enjoy a planned fruit snack

Here are some actions you can take to get this strategy working for you. On a sheet of paper, write the five headings from the above mindless eating records across the top. Then, using information from your food diary, write down the triggers (the places, related activities, and emotions) in the corresponding columns. Start with either your home, work, or social environment. Decide if each trigger is just a bad habit or if it serves an emotional need, such as anxiety reducer, mood lifter, or social companion. If it is serving another emotional need, refer to our coping strategies in Chapter 5 for new ways to fill those needs. If it's just a bad habit, decide how to break the behavior chain of this trigger or change any link that leads to eating. For example, Peter found himself stopping at the same fast-food restaurant because he passed it every night on the way home from work. To break this link, he started taking a different route home. Carl found that the bowl of peanut M&M's in his living room was too much to handle. He replaced them with individually wrapped 20-calorie Hershey's Tastetation candies. These strategies are simple, but they worked. Once you develop strategies for triggers in one setting, go on to tackle additional ones in other settings and repeat the process until you've combated all the triggers that cause you to lose control.

If you are unable to break certain triggers because they've become rituals in your life, then you may need some professional help. Some people have a lifelong struggle with their weight and are unable to gain control because of an underlying psychological problem that needs special attention. Binge eating disorder, or BED, is frequently associated with food rituals that are hard to break (see Chapter 8).

Success Boosters

Now that you're becoming a conscious consumer, you're keeping healthier alternatives readily available. You better understand your eating triggers and have been able to extinguish the main ones. You've also learned how drinking water can do much more than just quench your thirst. Check your progress with the following questions:

	Yes	No
■ Am I more aware of my mindless eating behaviors?	___	___
■ Am I making smarter choices?	___	___
■ Am I planning ahead so I have healthier alternatives more readily available?	___	___

- Have I been able to identify my eating triggers
  at home, work, and social events?   ____   ____
- Have I developed an action plan to tame my main
  eating triggers?   ____   ____
- Is my action plan working most of the time? ____   ____
- Am I drinking more water?   ____   ____
- Does my diary support my answers?   ____   ____

Hearty Portioner

Weight Busters
Pace Your Mind and Your Body

Hearty portioners are bred in America where small, medium, and large food portions have been replaced by large, family-size, and gigantic. Whether you're eating in a restaurant, picking up food through a drive-through, or fixing meals at home, the amount of food served in America has grown out of control. Typical hearty portioners talk about always finishing what's on their plates, not knowing when to stop eating, never quite feeling full until it's too late, and eating fast because they're always in a hurry. If your fast-paced life has you eating double-time, then this first strategy will help you to slow your pace and bring mindfulness, healthier portions, and less indigestion back to the dining table. You may be surprised to know that mindfulness and healthier portions are a twosome. Let me explain. When was the last time you wolfed down a serving of spinach or a sweet potato? And think about if you're ever able to savor slowly a serving of french fries? When you eat fast food, you tend to eat fast. As you bring mindfulness to the table, you'll not only find yourself eating less, but you'll also start gravitating toward making more conscious food choices, toward portions that satisfy rather than stuff, toward nutrition that fuels your body and mind.

Dietitian Dawn Jackson teaches her hearty portioner patients what she calls the "5 and 5 rule" to help them become more aware *in the moment*. Dawn explains that when people know what they "should" be doing but don't, it is *in the moment* that their decision power fails them. So she asks that 5 seconds before they eat, her patients remind themselves to eat slowly and enjoy their food. She teaches them that since the taste buds are in the mouth, once they swallow the fun is over, so it's better not to rush.

> ⤜ *Nibble on This* ⤛
> "Pace, don't race."
> —DAWN JACKSON, REGISTERED DIETITIAN, NORTHWESTERN MEMORIAL HOSPITAL WELLNESS INSTITUTE

Then, 5 minutes into the meal, Dawn tells patients to "put down the fork and push away," deciding *in the moment* how they feel and whether or not they're enjoying their food. By paying attention to your early signs of fullness, you will be more likely to stop eating way before you feel stuffed and uncomfortable.

Proportion Your Plate

This strategy allows you to eat less of your main course protein while indulging in more lower-calorie and fiber-rich vegetable, fruit, and whole-grain side dishes. Let me explain by using a typical picnic plate divided into three compartments—two smaller-sized nooks and one large compartment. If you are like most Americans, you grew up using the large compartment for hamburgers, hot dogs, chicken, and the like, while the two smaller areas may have been for vegetable, fruit, or starch side dishes such as corn, coleslaw, or potato salad. Your present challenge is to reproportion your plate by filling the large section of the plate with nutrient-rich vegetables, fruits, and salads and moving the meat portion and starch to the smaller nooks. The following table gives some examples of ways to do this, as do the recipes in Chapter 7. The beauty of this technique is that you don't have to give up anything—just relegate meat (or any other high-calorie foods) to the level of a supporting actor—not the romantic lead.

Proportioning Your Plate

Old Proportions	New Healthier Proportions
3 pieces of chicken, small side salad, mashed potatoes	Large entrée salad with grilled chicken strips, and whole-grain bread
Deep-fried shrimp and french fries	Whole wheat pasta with shrimp and vegetables
12-ounce steak, baked potato, and broccoli	4-ounce steak and vegetable stir fry over brown rice
Double cheeseburger and chips	Veggie burger on whole wheat bun, with lettuce, tomato, pickle; three-bean salad

Other ideas for following this strategy are to develop a 2-to-1 ratio when serving yourself at home: 2 portions of the vegetable or salad side dish for 1 portion of the main course protein. If you go for seconds, choose more of the side dishes (vegetables, salads, soups) instead of more main course. When eating in restaurants, take home half of your meat or main course portion, and ask for extra vegetables or salad. When eating family style in ethnic restaurants, choose at least one vegetarian entrée. Ethnic restaurants typically have a variety of vegetable-based dishes or dishes with these healthier proportions. In addition, they have more choices that contain plant-based protein sources such as tofu or beans. And last, pay attention to how you feel after eating a less-protein-heavy meal. Many people say that they feel more comfortable, have more energy, and are more satisfied—in essence, they enjoy being able to eat larger volumes of food without feeling overstuffed.

Be Savvy about Servings

Most hearty portioners don't have any sense of a healthy food portion. If that's also you, you're certainly not to blame since you have faithfully kept up your end of the bargain—given more food to eat, more food is eaten. This occurs because your visual senses override your internal signaling. For example, in one study of snack foods, people ate more M&M's from a two-pound bag than from a one-pound bag and more popcorn from a jumbo container than from a medium container.

> ⮞ *Nibble on This* ⮜
> Studies show that the more food you're given, the more food you eat.

To put this strategy into action, I want you to start paying more attention to food labels—particularly to the calories per serving sizes, which is more important than a product's carbohydrate, fat, or protein contents. If you look only at the calories on a label without also reading its serving size, you're missing the main point when it comes to weight loss.

To apply this strategy to yourself, you need to pay attention to the portion sizes of your typical meals and snacks and, using the food labels or the standard serving sizes in Chapter 2, identify the types of foods you are overeating. Foods my patients commonly identify are cereal (some eat 2 cups instead of 1 cup), pasta (some eat 3 cups instead of 1 cup—that is, two ½-cup servings), meat (some eat 8–10 ounces instead of 3–4 ounces), and ice cream (some eat 1½ cups instead of ½ cup). Some of my patients find that measuring their 1 cup of cereal each morning keeps them in better control. It helps others to divide their bulk purchases of chicken, fish, and meat into individual portions the size of a deck of cards or a cassette—ready for freezing. Still others consciously take a smaller serving of pasta but then fill up on the lower-calorie, stir-fry vegetables.

Many of my patients turn to portion-controlled products such as Healthy Choice, Lean Cuisine, and Weight Watchers Smart Ones frozen entrées for an easy and quick meal during their busy workweeks.

> ⮞ *Nibble on This* ⮜
> Eating portion-controlled frozen entrées helps to recalibrate your eyes and stomach.

If you're still hungry, add a side salad with roasted soy nuts or dried apricots to the meal. Drinking more water is also helpful. But remember that for this strategy to work, as you're eating smaller portions of some foods, you're fill-ing up on low-calorie fruits and vegetables—so you don't go hungry. Single wrapped or bagged servings of snacks and desserts, like string cheese, fat-free pudding cups, and low-fat granola bars, help hearty portioners as well. Take Andrea, who instead of opening a package of cookies—with no end in sight—now bakes one single serving of frozen cookie dough and enjoys a 180 calorie hot, chewy treat.

Using smaller plates and bowls is another strategy that improves visual cueing. At home, consider downsizing to 10-inch plates instead of 12-inch ones and using smaller cereal bowls instead of large ones. Climb on the stepstool so you can reach the special guest dinnerware you haven't used in 5 years. Eat off smaller but prettier plates and bowls. This will perk you up. Some of my patients have even switched to smaller wineglasses. If you tra-ditionally eat family style, serving individual plates of food from the stove will reduce the likelihood of taking second and third helpings of food.

This tactic worked wonderfully for Tanya who struggled to keep the family's dinner portions under control. By age 30, Tanya's weight had creeped up to over 200 pounds. As she realized that her husband and two children were also gaining weight, she found that their family-style dining was their undoing. So she began setting the table with reproportioned (and smaller) meal plates, which Tanya herself would dish out. Anyone who wanted seconds had to get up from the table and serve himself or herself, which meant thinking twice about whether he or she was still hungry for more. Having fewer dirty serving platters to clean up was another benefit. Tanya also made a special effort to prepare extra vegetable and fruit side dishes to accompany leaner cuts of meat and chicken. Over several weeks, the family made a painless transition from hearty portioners to healthy por-tioners.

Overcome Portion Traps

Your new awareness about portion sizes will help you to combat the hidden portion traps when eating out. Even so, it's so easy to fall prey to them that it's important to arm yourself with a plan of action. The following table suggests some good strategies.

Dining Out Portion Traps

Portion Trap	Plan of Action
Unlimited rolls, bread, and butter	Ask waitress not to bring rolls to table, bring rolls at same time as dinner, place one roll on plate, eat rolls dry, don't refill the bread basket.
Alcohol	Limit to one and drink slowly, try nonalcoholic drinks, switch to calorie-free soft drinks or water.
Salad dressings	Always ask for dressing on the side, use tines of fork to evenly distribute over salad, ask for low-fat or fat-free dressings.
Pasta	Order half serving, split entrée, or take half home.
Meat or entrée	Order half-serving, split entrée, or take half home.
Dessert	Always share, try one dessert for the table, order berries or other fresh fruit, or decline altogether.

Anticipating these portion traps is really half of the battle. The other half is making sure that you're choosing more salad, vegetable, and fruit dishes so you don't go hungry. "Meat and potatoes" eaters find this strategy particularly helpful once they get into the habit of ordering a side salad and asking for the vegetable of the day.

Hearty portioners also need to know how to navigate probably the biggest portion trap around, buffet-style eating, where indulgence is the expected route to take—unless you have a plan.

> ### ➤ *Nibble on This* ⬉
> When you devise a plan to beat the buffet, you have something besides willpower to depend on.

My patients find the following strategies helpful:

■ Walk around the entire buffet before selecting, so you can prioritize your healthy favorites rather than piling on food after food after food.

- Use the smallest plate, preferably a salad-size one, to give you instant portion and calorie control. Sure, you can keep going back for seconds and thirds, but you're usually more mindful when you have to get up, walk to the table, and serve yourself again.
- Choose foods that bring you pleasure and good nutrition, such as specialty salads, grilled vegetables, and/or delicious fresh fruit—a fiber-filled nutritionist's dream. As long as you pass on the salads covered in mayonnaise or creamy dressings, you usually can't go wrong. If a carving station showcases lean meats, or if seafood is available, treat yourself to a small portion.
- Proportion your plate so that three-quarters is covered with fruits, vegetables, and whole grains, and no more than one-quarter is covered with protein.
- You can try planning for a buffet meal by eating less during the day. However, this method can backfire if you become so ravenous that you are sure to overeat. Try this strategy once and see if it works for you.
- If you desire, savor a small amount of a favorite food, often found on the dessert table: Chocolate-covered strawberries, cake with fresh berries, or a taffy apple can all satisfy your sweet tooth with the balance of nutritious fruit. Or enjoy a bite or two of apple pie, a cookie, or a brownie. Remember—there are no forbidden foods.
- Always enjoy the moment, the people you're with, and the event itself. And if there's dancing, by all means, join in.

Success Boosters

As you're eating smaller portions of food (and also filling up on lower-calorie fruits and vegetables so you don't go hungry), you're feeling more satisfied, more energetic—and less stuffed after eating. You're enjoying your slower pace of eating, both inside and outside the home. You're more portion savvy and regularly practice strategies for overcoming portion traps when dining out. Continue to monitor your success with these questions:

	Yes	No
- Am I eating smaller portions (and feeling less stuffed after eating)?	___	___

	Yes	No
■ Am I eating more slowly?	____	____
■ Am I enjoying my slower-paced meals more?	____	____
■ Am I thinking about the picnic plate to reproportion my plate?	____	____
■ Am I using the food label calories per serving size to make smarter food choices?	____	____
■ Have I tried calorie-controlled meals to retrain my eyes and stomach?	____	____
■ Have I found snack foods that come in single-serving sizes that I enjoy?	____	____
■ Have I downsized my dinnerware at home?	____	____
■ Am I avoiding portion traps when eating out?	____	____
■ Am I following my "beat the buffet" plan?	____	____

Deprived Sneaker

Weight Busters
Dismiss "Cheating"

Some patients talk about being "good" with their diet one week or "cheating" another week, a common dieting mind-set you need to break early on because it actually does the opposite of what you're trying to achieve. Instead of strengthening a patient's confidence and determination, it feeds your feelings of guilt and powerlessness. Nowhere is this more evident than with deprived sneakers who complain of feeling guilty when they overeat yet deprived when they eat and who just never seem satisfied.

The first step is to embrace *all* food. My program is very different than other extreme diets you may have been on in the past, such as the grapefruit diet or the high-protein diet, with long lists of forbidden foods. My program in contrast allows all foods—within moderation. Without the expected lists of "good" and "bad" foods or silly food rules to follow, you realize that perfection is not the name of the game. Instead, through the process of learning what you're doing and why, you are able to figure out ways to avoid overeating in certain situations. Rather than focusing on feeling guilty and beating yourself up, you learn to focus on the process and how to do better the next time.

Add Satisfaction with Fat and Fiber

Some people have mood swings. Deprived sneakers have swings in their dietary habits—from severely restricted eating to overindulging. Heart-healthy fat and fiber seem to center their pendulums.

If you're a deprived sneaker, just the thought of adding some fat to your diet can be hard at first because you know that this adds calories. But because the added fat will make your tasteless "diet" foods taste better and because fat makes you feel full longer, you'll feel more satiated and be less inclined to overindulge later on—and that means fewer calories overall.

> ⪼ *Nibble on This* ⪻
>
> Eat "heart-healthy fats" to satisfy your taste buds without draining your health.

The point is to use fat and fiber to bring pleasure and health to your table. Since everyone has different tastes and preferences, you'll need to try different products until you find ones you truly enjoy. This strategy may mean eating fewer fat-free foods and instead looking for reduced-fat products that may taste better. Or it may mean using olive oil when stir-frying instead of cooking with nonfat cooking spray only. For still another person, it may mean enjoying other heart-healthy fats: a handful of peanuts in stir-fry dishes or some avocado in salads. The following table gives you ways to replace your traditional "diet" fare with more satisfying and healthy alternatives.

Satisfying Alternatives

Traditional "Diet" Foods	More Satisfying Alternatives (with added fat and fiber)
Breakfast	
English muffin and diet margarine	High-fiber bagel with light cream cheese and tomato slices
Lunch	
Salad with fat-free dressing and dry cracker	Salad with reduced-fat dressing, grilled chicken, soy nuts, and high-fiber crispbread

Satisfying Alternatives *(cont.)*

Traditional "Diet" Foods	More Satisfying Alternatives (with added fat and fiber)
Dinner	
Leanest Boca Burger without bun or condiments	Boca Burger (with the most fat) on whole-grain bun with barbecue sauce, pickle, and tomato slice; cup of bean soup
Snacks	
Fat-free cookie	Cookie with fiber (try Natural Ovens brand)
Fat-free yogurt	Reduced-fat yogurt with dried fruit and nuts mixed in
Fat-free, sugar-free ice cream	Reduced-fat frozen yogurt or ice cream with fresh berries

As you focus on adding a variety of fiber-filled foods to your meals and snacks, remember to drink extra water and pay attention to your changes in feelings of satisfaction. Since it's common for deprived sneakers to have their "safe" lunches that they rarely deviate from, try surprising your taste buds once in a while with some new meal ideas. Norma discovered the versatility of different foods, like baby spinach—which made a hearty lunch on a high-fiber bagel with Light Laughing Cow cheese and sliced tomatoes or even a delicious entrée salad topped with grilled salmon. Bulk or bagged baby spinach became a regular item on her weekly shopping list. Norma also discovered microwave bean soups that were loaded with fiber—sometimes up to 14 grams per serving. These tasted great with whole-grain bread for a filling, last-minute lunch or dinner. As you try new foods, see if fiber can combine with heart-healthy fats to increase your dining satisfaction.

Moderate Your Sweet Tooth

Since it's common for deprived sneakers to still have cravings for their favorite dessert-type foods, learning moderation is key. Here I suggest the 80/20 rule: If 80 percent of your diet is healthy, then it's okay if 20 percent is less healthy. Many experts use this rule to give patients a better idea of how to realistically enjoy a healthy diet.

But this strategy takes some practice. Here's what you need to do. Once

you're already eating meals that bring you more satisfaction, choose preportioned desserts, when possible. Some patient favorites are 140-calorie Diana's
Bananas Banana Babies (chocolate-dipped frozen bananas) and 140-calorie
Silhouette Ice Cream Sandwiches. Since you can't always find preportioned
snacks, try controlling your portions using downsized dinnerware at
home—custard-size bowls instead of cereal bowls for reduced-fat ice cream
or frozen yogurt. Or use a 50-calorie waffle bowl (by Keebler) to give your
frozen dessert or low-fat pudding more eye appeal and taste—and fiber
when topped with fresh raspberries. Using the 80/20 rule, you can savor
these sweet foods without guilt.

Socialize and Enjoy

Most deprived sneakers have developed two eating styles—the one they
show in public and the one they do in private. The "public" showing is typically composed of eating only healthy and calorie-controlled foods. If
higher-calorie or "sinful" food is served, it's usually only picked at or
avoided entirely. This pattern is in stark contrast to the "private" eating,
where rules are abandoned and favorite foods are savored. This long-held
pattern of "good girl" and "bad girl" continues to foster internal conflicts
and out-of-control body weight. The first step to break this emotional
merry-go-round is to break down the two self-imposed eating styles.

Allowing yourself to enjoy previously forbidden foods in social situations is an important therapeutic step for the deprived sneaker. Ask yourself
what you really feel like eating and order it. Enjoy and savor each bite, eating
slowly and paying attention to aroma, temperature, flavor, texture, and fullness. Ask yourself how much you are enjoying it and give yourself permission to stop eating whenever you want—you don't have to finish what is in
front of you. If done successfully, it will rid your urge to self-indulge when
no one is around.

Success Boosters

Whether alone or in a group, you're feeling less guilt and more pleasure at
mealtimes. Adding fat and fiber has helped to make your meals more satisfying. And you've been practicing ways to moderate your sweet tooth. Monitor your progress with these questions:

	Yes	No
■ Am I feeling less guilt and more pleasure at mealtimes?	___	___
■ Have I stopped talking about "cheating" on my diet?	___	___
■ Am I eating more foods with healthy fats and fiber?	___	___
■ Am I feeling more satisfied when I eat?	___	___
■ Am I practicing moderation when it comes to eating sweets?	___	___
■ Are my "private" and "public" eating patterns becoming more similar?	___	___
■ Am I looking forward to social situations as opportunities to meet more people with common interests?	___	___

Making a Move

Now that you've brought new structure and foods to the table, it's time to make a move. Whether you've been in an exercise rut or even completely sedentary because you feel unmotivated, overwhelmed, or uninspired, the next chapter is for you.

■   ■   ■   ■   ■

Chapter 4

Shaping Your Exercise Personality

■ ■ ■ ■ **B** ecoming more active is a given if you want to lose weight. But the strategies I recommend for successfully doing so differ depending on your exercise pattern profile. While some of you need strategies to combat your less active lifestyle (which can also feed feelings of exhaustion, low energy, stiffness, being out of shape, and feeling older than you are), others need to know how to step up their programs. Knowing what works and what doesn't for different personality types has helped me develop specific strategies to get each of you started—and keep you going.

Hate-to-Move Struggler

Weight Busters
Count All Activity
Being more active may conjure up unpleasant thoughts of sweating and exhaustion. You'll quickly learn, however, that it doesn't have to be that hard. There really are easier ways to be physically active (and healthier) without having to join a health club or even learn a new sport. Try these natural fitness tips to sneak in more activity—without drastically changing your routine or having to make a huge time commitment.

- Take the stairs instead of the elevator.
- Park your car farther away from your destination.
- Get off the bus or train one stop earlier and walk.
- Walk up and down escalators.

- Take longer routes when shopping.
- Walk to coworker's office instead of E-mailing.
- Convert coffee breaks into walking breaks.
- Pace while talking on phone (using cordless phone or long handset cord).
- Take a walk while waiting at the airport or for an appointment.
- Walk to the store or to mail letters.
- Walk once around the mall before you shop.
- When unloading groceries from your car, carry one bag at a time into the house.
- Walk your baby longer when out in the stroller.
- Walk your child to school.
- Walk your dog longer.
- Hide your television remote control.
- Work in your garden (mowing, raking, weeding, digging, etc.).
- Shovel snow.
- Wash your own car.
- Do your own housework (scrubbing, mopping, dusting, polishing, etc.).
- When carrying laundry upstairs, make several trips instead of one.

Instead of needing hours to drive to and from a health club, change clothes, work out, and shower, I'm talking about accumulating activity throughout your normal day, just the way Bill did. He allowed 15 more minutes in the morning for parking his car farther away from his office and walking up the stairs instead of taking the elevator and another 15 minutes at the end of the day for the return trip. Instead of going to the nearest bus stop after work, Suzanne walked as long as she could and caught the same bus but farther down the route. This strategy allowed her to unwind after work and get in 30 minutes of activity along the way. For Natalie, walking her dog farther in the mornings, afternoons, and evenings became her easy way to add activity to her routine. (Her dog is slimmer, healthier, and happier too.)

Try clipping a pedometer to your belt or waistband to measure how many steps you take just doing activities of daily living (ADLs). As pedometers motivate you to keep moving, they also give you an objective way to track your progress. At the same time, they can help to change your self-image from someone who hates to exercise to someone who values being active and understands its health benefits. If you already purchased a pedometer for the three-week starter plan, it's time to start wearing it again. If you don't have one, now's the time to get one and follow these pedometer basics.

Pedometer Basics	
Purpose	By counting the number of steps you take each day, a pedometer makes activity fun and gives you an objective way to mark your progress.
How to Purchase	Buy one that counts steps, not miles. Most sporting goods stores carry them for under $30. Or you can order the Digi-Walker #AE120 from Accusplit in San Jose, California, 1-800-935-1996, ext. 204; www.accusplit.com.
How to Record Baseline Activity	Use your pedometer to record the number of steps taken per day for 2 to 3 days (preferably a weekday and a weekend day). Calculate and record your average baseline.
How to Track Steps	On a separate piece of paper, write the days of the week along with the steps taken each day. Weekly, calculate and record your average steps taken.
How to Set Goals	Set a goal for yourself to increase the number of steps or distance week to week by 10 percent. For example, if your daily baseline averages 4,000 steps the first week, then your goal is to increase the second week to 4,400 (an increase of 400 steps daily) and to 4,840 the third week.

Alternatively, simply increase your ADLs and note the number of additional steps taken.

We established the 10,000 Step Club in our program at Northwestern as an incentive for patients to increase ADLs. Depending on your stride, 10,000 steps equates to about 3 to 5 miles, which is a realistic longer-term goal that many strugglers can safely achieve, some within 2 to 3 months, others within 4 to 5 months. Remember that the goal is safe progress (using the 10 percent guideline above), not perfection. The beauty of this strategy is that you can significantly increase your activity level without having to join a formal exercise program.

➣ Nibble on This ⇐

On average, inactive people take 2,000 to 4,000 steps per day, moderately active people take 5,000 to 7,000 steps per day, and active people take 10,000 or more steps per day.

Tim took this challenge to heart, once he realized that being more active at work didn't require time off or fancy exercise equipment, just a little creativity. His solution was to purchase an extralong headset cord that permitted him to pace while talking on the phone in his office. By introducing this "ingenious invention" (Tim's description), he was able to add 500 steps each day while performing the same job. (I didn't have the heart to tell Tim that cordless phones were already invented for the same reason.)

Energize Your Body and Mind

Though strugglers often identify with low-energy descriptions such as feeling tired, fatigued, exhausted, sleepy, worn out, beat, and/or disinterested in sex, they initially don't realize that these problems are all exacerbated by their sedentary lifestyle. But once strugglers start wearing their pedometers and maximizing their daily activities, they become energized naturally as a consequence of being more active.

Some people benefit from thinking about how their energy level shifts as they become more active. Making this connection between your inactivity and feelings of low energy (and conversely your activity and feelings of high energy) is sure to move you forward in this program. Energy walks (brisk 5–10 minute walks when you're tired or stressed) can reduce tension, improve mood, and energize you—particularly at your low-energy or stressful times of day.

> ⤳ *Nibble on This* ⬳
>
> Just 10 minutes of brisk walking can give you an hour or two of increased energy.

Find Fun

Once you know that being active doesn't have to be uncomfortable or boring (and can even have positive effects on your life), it's time to pick up the pace and your enjoyment. If your typical weeknight activities are watching TV, surfing the Net, or reading, and your weekend activities are dining out and seeing a movie, I recommend that you change your routine and set a new course, picking from dozens of social and enjoyable activities: miniature golf, bowling, walking through the zoo or park, dancing, apple picking, kite flying, bike riding, golfing, tennis, dancing, swimming, playing Ping-Pong, hiking, shooting baskets, playing softball, canoeing, cross-country skiing, ice skating, snowshoeing, or sledding. A good way to begin is to make a list of *active* leisuretime activities in or around your neighborhood that you could see yourself doing. Your specific activities will vary with the seasons, your time commitment, and of course your budget, but certainly finding fun can be a year-round event.

> ❧ *Nibble on This* ❧
> Active leisure is not an oxymoron.

Sara took my advice. Family television time and watching rented videos were replaced with family walks in the park, bike riding, shooting baskets, and playing catch in their front yard. Instead of being resistant, Sara's family seized on her initiative to change their long-standing couch potato behavior. They all knew that lying around wasn't particularly good for them, but nobody took the lead to make any changes. Of course they still rent movies and watch TV together, but now these are relegated to their less common family activities.

Buddy Up

For many people, it's more fun to do activities with friends and others than to do them alone, especially for strugglers who have a million excuses for not being active. If support and accountability will make it more likely that you'll do a particular activity (such as going for a half-hour walk or bike ride), then find yourself a partner. This could be a walking buddy, a fellow dancer, a golfing friend, a night bowling league, an exercise trainer, or even your dog. Or it could even be a casual acquaintance that you meet through taking a tennis class. In addition, many cities have clubs or buddy groups for like-minded people who enjoy walking, cycling, cross-country skiing, or even kayaking.

> ⤜ *Nibble on This* ⤛
>
> When it comes to exercise, peer pressure can be both healthy and motivating.

The buddy up strategy is easy to carry out, once you know your daily schedule, the supportive people in your life, and the activities available in your community. In Sara's case above, she buddied up with her own family members. Another patient buddied up with her spouse for nightly after-dinner walks. Without the distraction of the television set or their barking dogs, this couple was able to connect with each other while briskly walking and winding down after their day's work. They liked their nightly outings so much that when the weather turned cold, they joined a local community center with an indoor track. Another struggler met a neighbor for 6 A.M. power walks 3 times a week. This patient knew he had to schedule his exercise time before work if he wanted to be successful. After receiving an exercise bike along with a one-hour in-home exercise trainer as a birthday gift, another struggler decided that buddying up with a professional was the best way for him to go. For the first time in his life, he didn't struggle with exercise the way he had in the past because the trainer was so motivating. After just six lessons, this patient had an in-home routine that was manageable, safe, and energizing.

Once you take a look at how much time you can commit, along with the people and programs available in your community, you can try buddying up. And remember that if your exercise buddy moves away or loses motivation, this doesn't mean that your program has to also stop. You just need to find another buddy.

Success Boosters

As you experience the painless ways to build activity into your lifestyle, you're feeling more energetic and more in control. You know that activity can be fun and energizing, especially when you buddy up. Check your progress with these questions:

	Yes	No
■ Am I counting all activity, including my ADLs?	____	____
■ Am I wearing a pedometer to track my activity?	____	____
■ Am I getting closer to reaching the 10,000 Step Club?	____	____
■ Am I paying attention to how my energy level varies with my activity?	____	____
■ Do "energy walks" give me an energy boost when I'm tired?	____	____
■ Am I trying more fun, leisuretime activities?	____	____
■ Have I found an activity buddy?	____	____

Self-Conscious Hider

Weight Busters
Dress the Part

After trying to better understand self-conscious hiders, I concluded that they needed to be more comfortable with themselves before they could even think or talk about exercising. To help these patients, I asked them what clothes feel comfortable and loose-fitting. I helped them banish their hidden association of exercise with spandex body-hugging clothes and replace that with the more real image of working out in clothes that they can move more easily in.

To dress the part, choose clothes with comfort in mind—comfortable to perform the workout and comfortable to be in around others. Pick a fabric that absorbs sweat and keeps you cool—like cotton. Women find that a good sports bra is essential, as are a good pair of shoes. And if you've been wearing the same ten-year-old gym shoes, it's time to splurge and buy yourself a new pair of athletic shoes to match your activity, such as walking or cross training. For active women's wear, sizes 14–40, call Junonia at 1-800-586-6642 for a free catalog.

Break a Sweat at Home

With comfort and security being an initial priority for self-conscious hiders, home is clearly their most safe and secure place for exercising. Add in that it's convenient, private, personalized, and time-saving, and it's the ideal atmosphere for hiders who would rather have fun while moving their bodies instead of worrying about how they look to others.

> ⮞ *Nibble on This* ⮜
>
> Your ideal workout spot may be the one in which you feel most at home.

Now that you've decided to break a sweat at home, you've got to choose your activity. Use the following suggestions as you work through your many choices:

- Powerhouse cleaning refers to cleaning continuously and at a quick pace so that you get a better workout. Some people find that multitasking their exercise and housecleaning is a win-win situation as they save money on cleaning help while also being more active.
- Exercise videos are a simple, cheap, and easy way to break a sweat at home. Just choose your favorite exercise guru (Denise Austin, Kathy Smith, Gin Miller, Richard Simmons) and workout routine (low-impact or step aerobics, dancing) and turn on the video recorder. Whether it's 15 minutes or an hour, it's all done in the privacy of your own home on your own schedule. For a free exercise video catalog, call Collage Video at 1-800-433-6769.
- If you want to step up to aerobic exercise equipment, it is important to select equipment that you can picture yourself using and enjoying for months and years to come. If you like walking, then a treadmill makes the most sense. If, however, you like bicycle riding or have physical limitations that prevent you from walking, then a stationary bike (upright or recumbent) is your best bet. Both machines allow you to burn calories while giving you a good aerobic workout. As for which brand to buy, this depends on cost, durability, and value, and for treadmills, whether you

want a motorized or nonmotorized model. For a higher-level workout, check out step machines or elliptical trainers. And for all machines, be sure that you have adequate space at home and that the equipment will support your body weight, and see if the store offers free in-home training for safety purposes. Since it's ideal to visit the showroom and actually try out the machine before you purchase it, remember to don your gym shoes and comfortable clothes. Before you rule out this option as too expensive, check your yellow pages for used exercise equipment stores or visit your local Salvation Army. One friend picked up a recumbent bike secondhand in perfect condition for $40.

■ For resistance training, you can select from a wide range of equipment depending on cost, versatility, and the space available in your home (both width and ceiling height). One of the easiest and cheapest ways to start is by buying resistance bands and hand weights. Or step up to barbells or even a multipurpose weight machine. Once again, check the machine's weight rating (the number of pounds it can support) to make sure it is safe for your size. With safety in mind, I recommend that you consult with a personal trainer or a resistance training book or video that covers the basics.

■ Think carefully about where to place the equipment. In addition to leaving enough room around the equipment to extend your arms and legs, you want to ensure that your "workout room" is as inviting as possible. Likewise, the time may go by quicker if you have a TV or radio in the room. Or place the treadmill overlooking a picture window so that natural sunlight enters the room.

> ⋑ *Nibble on This* ⋐

"Unless we exercise the muscles we have, properly, we lose 5–7 pounds of muscle tissue every decade of adult life. Because muscles are the engines of the body, this is similar to dropping from an 8-cylinder car, to a 6-cylinder car, to a 4-cylinder car, to a motor scooter."

—Dr. Wayne L. Westcott and Dr. Thomas R. Baechle, *Strength Training Past 50*

Be Inconspicuous

Self-conscious hiders do not like being active around others—period. Their reasons vary and can be quite distressing, such as being embarrassed of their body, painfully aware that they have difficulty bending and moving the same way as others (such as unable to get up from a sitting position on the floor, getting flushed and sweaty after any activity), and unsure if a particular machine will safely hold their weight. But this doesn't mean that being active at home is your only option. Instead hiders can become inconspicuous exercisers by choosing their activity and environment wisely.

First I recommend that you build activity naturally into your routine. Doing your own gardening, washing your own car, power shopping through the grocery store aisles, and walking your baby longer in the stroller are ways you can remain inconspicuous while staying active. Or commit to a walking program, which can be done practically anywhere, anytime, at any pace, and with anybody. You're inconspicuous because you're joining the masses of individuals doing the same thing, whether it's along the lakefront or river walk, through forest paths, on city streets, or on neighborhood sidewalks.

If you want to work out in a health club, you may feel more comfortable doing so once you've had success breaking a sweat at home. Some people like joining a health club that specifically caters to special populations, such as Women's Workout World. Others want a health club that offers times, classes, and equipment they find convenient and still comfortable. You can be inconspicuous in a low-impact aerobics class geared for beginners or pick workout times when your health club is less busy—such as midmorning, after lunch, before 3:00, or even after 8 P.M.

Move and Meditate

This last strategy turns your attention while exercising from being outwardly conscious to inwardly mindful, which helps you in several ways. First, it allows you to relax your mind and body long enough to reach that ultimate state of mind—what some people call the endorphin rush or a runner's high. Second, it encourages you to clear your mind of the day's stress so exercise itself becomes a tension releaser.

> ⇝ *Nibble on This* ⇜
> Exercise is as much for the mind as it is for the body.

Try to focus your thoughts and feelings on your active body—that is, the depth and rhythm of your breathing, the tension and relaxation of your muscles, the warmth and moisture of your skin. As you forget about your troubles, enjoy the quietness in your mind that exercise can bring. People find different techniques helpful for eliciting relaxation while exercising. Some focus on the repetitive rhythms of their breath, moving feet, or swim strokes. Others repeat a word (such as "calm") to focus their thoughts on the present moment. If you find yourself thinking about having to go to the grocery store or an upcoming meeting, acknowledge these thoughts but then quickly let them go. Once you reach that higher level of exercise that brings an elevated mood and improved self-image, you will no longer feel the need self-consciously to hide your healthy and active body.

Success Boosters
You're feeling more comfortable breaking a sweat at home and even increasing your ADLs in public. With an increased feeling of security, both your mind and body are better able to appreciate the many benefits that exercise brings. Check your progress with these questions:

	Yes	No
■ Am I wearing comfortable, loose-fitting clothes while exercising?	____	____
■ Do I have a good-fitting pair of athletic shoes?	____	____
■ Am I breaking a sweat at home?	____	____
■ Am I becoming an inconspicuous exerciser outside of my home?	____	____
■ Am I becoming less outwardly self-conscious of my body?	____	____
■ Am I becoming more inwardly mindful as I exercise?	____	____
■ Am I enjoying exercise more?	____	____

Inexperienced Novice

Weight Busters
Ease into Stretching

Inexperienced novices don't know what to do first. I recommend starting with an important part of physical activity that has been shown to release tension, increase range of motion, decrease muscle soreness and stiffness, prevent injury, maintain flexibility, and feel good—a regular stretching program.

> ➤ *Nibble on This* ➤
>
> "Don't stretch to be flexible or to see how far you can go. Stretch to feel good."
>
> —BOB ANDERSON, *STRETCHING*

As you stretch different parts of the body, it can be a wonderful way to connect your body and mind as you develop a new kind of body awareness. Stretching is the easiest of the physical activity components to do as long as you understand these guidelines.

- *Do* breathe naturally while stretching.
- *Do* hold your stretches to the point of gentle tension for 10–30 seconds.
- *Don't* bounce.
- *Don't* overstretch to the point of pain.

Getting started can be as easy as taking a few extra minutes first thing in the morning. In fact, I recommend that you become familiar with what I call the "stretches of daily living" or SDLs.

- Try lying-down SDLs in the morning and at night before you go to sleep. (Note: Stretch on a firm—but not hard—surface like a soft rug or a firm mat.)
- Try sitting SDLs when working at the computer, sitting in your office chair, or stopped at a red light in your car.

■ Try standing SDLs while using the copy machine at work, filling your car up with gas, waiting in line at the grocery store, or standing at a bus stop.

SDLs (Stretches of Daily Living)

Position	Stretches
Lying Down On Your Back	**Lying knee hug:** Bend one knee and clasp both hands behind your thigh and pull gently toward your chest. Hold for 10–15 seconds. Keep the other leg as straight as possible without locking your knee. Keep your lower back flat against the mat or rug. Repeat 2 times for both legs. **Total body elongation stretch:** Stretch your arms above your head and extend your fingers and then point your toes as you stretch your legs. Hold for 5 seconds and then relax. Repeat 2 times.
Sitting	**Shoulder shrugs:** Raise your shoulders upward toward your ears. When you feel a slight tension, hold for 5 seconds. Then relax your shoulders. Repeat 2 times. **Arms above head stretch:** With your arms stretched up above your head, interlock your fingers and turn your palms so they're facing upward. Hold for 10–15 seconds and relax. Repeat 2 times.
Standing	**Standing calf stretch:** Stand with your hands on your hips and one foot in front of the other. Bend your front leg to stretch the calf muscle of your rear leg, keeping both heels flat on the ground and your toes pointing straight ahead. When you feel gentle tension in the calf muscle, hold the position for 10–15 seconds. Repeat on other side. **Standing quad stretch:** Stand and bend your right knee, grasping that ankle with your right hand. Hold a gentle stretch for 10–15 seconds without arching your back. Some people feel more balanced with the idle hand touching the wall. Repeat on other side.

Though an essential part of physical activity, stretching does not replace aerobics or strength training. In contrast, stretching warms up your muscles and gets them ready to work. In addition, many experts suggest that you warm your muscles by marching in place or walking and swinging your arms for a few minutes before stretching. By stretching warm muscles *before* and *after* your planned activity you will be able to advance your exercise program with more success and without fear of muscle soreness or injury.

These stretching exercises relax you and help your body to feel and work better. Stretches will give you a new kind of awareness of and control over your body. Since on some days your muscles are tighter than on other days, you need to be sensitive to these changes, listen to your body, and hold only the stretches that feel comfortable.

Exercise Stretches for Aerobic or Resistance Training

Standing arms above head stretch: With your arms stretched above your head, interlock your fingers and turn your palms so they face upward. Hold for 10–15 seconds and relax. Repeat 2 times.

Standing triceps stretch: With your arms above your head, hold the elbow of one arm with the other hand so the elbow is pointing toward the ceiling. Gently pull the elbow and hold for 10–15 seconds. Repeat with your other arm.

Standing calf stretch: Stand with hands on hips and both feet on the floor, one in front of the other. Bend front leg to stretch calf muscle of rear leg, keeping both heels flat on the ground and toes pointing straight ahead. When you feel gentle tension in calf muscle, hold position for 10–15 seconds. Repeat on other side.

Standing quad stretch: Stand and bend your right knee, grasping your ankle with your right hand. Hold gentle stretch for 10–15 seconds without arching your back. Some people feel more balanced using their opposite hand to touch the wall. Repeat on other side.

Sitting groin stretch: Sit on the floor with the soles of your feet together and gently hold on to your toes. Bending at the hips, gently pull yourself forward. Hold for 10–15 seconds.

Sitting hamstring stretch: Sit with one leg bent while keeping the other leg stretched out about 45° to the side. Bend forward slowly from the hip toward the straight leg, while keeping your head upright. Hold for 10–15 seconds. Repeat on the other side.

Lying knee hug: Lie flat on your back. Bend one knee and clasp both hands behind your thigh and pull gently toward your chest. Hold for 10–15 seconds. Keep the other leg as straight as possible without locking your knee. Keep your lower back flat against the mat or rug. Repeat 3 times for both legs.

Lying hamstring stretch: Lie on your back with both knees bent and feet on floor. Clasp both hands behind your right thigh and gently pull the leg toward your chest until you feel light tension in your hamstring. Hold for 10–15 seconds. Repeat 3 times for both legs. Keep your lower back flat against the floor.

*Don't worry if you can't pull your leg far (hamstring stretch) or bend over far (groin stretch). Stretch only as far as is comfortable for you. And as you exhale, you'll feel stretching or easing.

Start Smart

Novices have never learned the ABCs of how to exercise and feel awkward or unsafe around exercise equipment. It turns out that there really are ABCs to exercise, although these fundamentals go by the letters FITTE. Walking through the details of the FITTE principle will give you the confidence to begin your program.

Different from ADLs, exercises such as speed walking, jogging, biking, swimming, and tennis are planned, structured, and repetitive. The FITTE principle (which stands for *F*requency, *I*ntensity, *T*ime, *T*ype, and *E*njoyment) will help you take the "in" out of "inexperienced." Since I recommend that most novices initiate their exercise program with walking, I use walking in the table descriptions, but the FITTE principle can be applied to any kind of aerobic exercise.

FITTE Principle

Frequency   The number of times you will be walking each week. Aim for a minimum of twice a week and preferably 3–4 times a week to start (with a longer-term goal of daily fitness walking). If you can find the time to walk only once a week in the beginning, that's a start. But quickly increase that to 2 or more outings if you want to see results.

Intensity   The vigor or pace of your walking. If you want to build fitness, you need to exercise at a level that is challenging to your heart, lungs, and entire body. A good way to gauge that level of intensity is to rate the effort or strain you are experiencing while walking, in other words, how much you are exerting yourself. Use a subjective rating scale ranging from 0 to 10, where 0 = how you feel at rest and 10 = how you'd feel if you were working as hard as possible. You want to work at an exertion rating of 6 or 7, where you're walking as if you're late to catch a train or bus. Exercising at this level, you are breathing harder, have an elevated pulse rate, are sweating, and can still talk but only in broken-up phrases. Remember to warm up before and cool down after exercise to decrease your chances of injury. Simply march in place or ride an exercise bike for a few minutes to warm your muscles, stretch, and begin your workout by building your pace slowly. Taper your pace at the end of the workout so your heart rate returns to normal and then end by stretching your warm muscles.

Time   The duration of your walking. The *minimum* goal is to accumulate 30 minutes of fitness walking on the days that you exercise. If you can do it all in one 30-minute period, that's fine. It doesn't matter if you get it in first thing in the morning or after dinner. But you also have the option of doing short bouts that add up to 30 minutes, such as two 15-minute walking sessions in one day. The total number of calories burned is determined by how long you walk (duration) and how hard you walk (intensity).

Type   The kind or mode of activity you choose. Though I am suggesting that you start with fitness walking, you will want to try other aerobic activities over time to keep your mind and body challenged and motivated.

Enjoyment   Do exercises that you find fun. If you get bored with walking on a treadmill, try walking outdoors (or vice versa). Seek activities and exercise partners that make you look forward to your workouts.

A last note about proper nutrition and hydration as it relates to working out. If you work out in the morning, make sure to eat a light carbohydrate-containing meal or snack first, since your body will be low on fuel; eat half a banana or some yogurt. For workouts that last longer than an hour, I also recommend that you replenish your body's glycogen stores 30 minutes after exercise by consuming a light snack (like a sports drink or orange juice and whole wheat crackers). Some people eat half of their breakfast before and half after their morning workout. If you work out after dinner, I recommend that you wait at least 45 minutes to let your food digest. *Always* drink plenty of water before, during, and after your workout. And listen to your body. Though you may feel some fatigue immediately after a workout, you should recover and feel energized within 30 minutes or so. If instead you feel weak, dizzy, or lightheaded, you need to get direction from your physician and later a certified personal trainer.

Mark Your Progress

Self-monitoring your progress is especially important for novices who have little or no experience to draw from. A food, mood, and movement diary is ideal for tracking your ADLs or other planned activities. If you are starting a more structured exercise routine (like walking on a treadmill or riding an exercise bike), you may want to use a more detailed activity record sheet that allows you to track specific elements of the FITTE principle.

FITTE Activity Record

Week	Frequency	Intensity/ Perceived Exertion	Time (minutes)	Type	Enjoyment/ Comments
1–2	M, W, F	3.2 mph/5	20	Treadmill	Felt more energetic
3	M, W, F	3.5 mph/6	25	Treadmill	Higher speed getting easier; feeling less stressed at work

Connie used a similar record to track her progress on a home stationary bike. As the weeks passed, she gradually increased the frequency, intensity, and time on the bike, which along with her dietary changes put her on the road to improved health and weight loss. Yet instead of feeling proud of her accomplishments, she felt disappointed that her weight loss was less than she expected—given all the time and effort she expended on the bike. Although the 3.5 pound weight loss over the first month was actually quite reasonable, Connie was focused only on the scale and not on any other health benefits of being more physically active. After asking Connie to complete the last column of her activity record, she documented the following, which helped her to better appreciate her progress: "took an inch off my waist—blouse and skirt fitting looser," "definitely less tired in late afternoon," and "feel better about how I look and feel." Focusing on all the benefits of exercise keeps you motivated.

Another wonderful tool is a pedometer to measure the number of steps taken or the distance covered (see pages 90–91). This device helps you track your progress and set new goals. If you decide to use a pedometer to chart your progress, buy one that counts steps, not miles. Set a goal to increase the number of daily steps taken week to week by 10 percent.

Build Muscle

Novices commonly avoid resistance training because they were never taught how to do it properly, have no real experience using weight machines, and are unfamiliar with the benefits of adding weight lifting to their routine. The sooner you add this exercise element to your program, the earlier you see the rewards of total physical fitness.

> ➣ *Nibble on This* ⋲
>
> "Muscles have memory. The more you exercise, the more your body will adapt."
>
> —MICHELLE SANDSTROM, FITNESS INSTRUCTOR, WILMETTE PARK DISTRICT

The benefits of strength training are varied. By building stronger muscles, you will naturally increase your endurance, which means that everyday activities will become much easier for you. Through strength training, your body composition also shifts by dropping fat and gaining muscle, which becomes noticeable as you reduce one or two clothing sizes and tighten your belt.

When it comes to doing resistance training, it's not unusual for patients to consult with a personal trainer (at least once) so they can get started safely. I highly recommend this—especially for novices who may not realize the importance of using good technique to decrease their chances of injury. Here are some questions to ask a trainer:

- What's your academic training?
  Look for a BS or MS in a health-related field such as exercise physiology, kinesiology, exercise science, or athletic training.
- What kinds of certifications do you have?
  Look for certifications beyond their academic training such as CPR (cardiopulmonary resuscitation), ACSM (American College of Sports Medicine), NSCA (National Strength and Conditioning Association), NATA (National Athletic Trainers' Association), or ACE (American Council on Exercise).

- Do you have liability insurance?
- Do you have references from former clients?

If a personal trainer isn't in your budget, here are some resistance training basics for getting started.

Resistance-Training Basics

- Muscles are built by pushing, pulling, or lifting weights that you find hard to move. You need to work your muscles in order to build them.

- Pick a weight load that you can move for 8 to 12 repetitions (reps) to the point of muscle fatigue. If you can't do at least 8 reps, the weight is too heavy. If you can easily do more than 12 reps, the weight is too light.

- Learn proper form to decrease your chances of injury. A proper sitting posture includes feet being planted firmly on the floor with your knees at a right angle (short people may have to rest feet on stool), neck and shoulders relaxed, head up and looking forward, and abdominal muscles tightened. A proper standing pose includes feet shoulder width apart with toes pointing forward, knees relaxed and *never* locked, neck and shoulders relaxed, head up and looking forward, abdominal muscles tightened, and buttocks tucked under to avoid arching your back. Work out in front of a mirror so you can check your form periodically. Stop if you feel pain.

- Exercise muscle groups one at a time, starting with the major muscle groups (back, chest, legs, shoulders, abdominals) followed by the smaller groups (upper and lower arms, lower legs). Since your legs represent 60 percent of your muscle mass, working on leg muscles is essential.

- A typical program involves doing 2 sets of 8–12 reps for each weight routine, 2 or 3 times per week (but the number of sets can vary from 1 to 3, depending on your initial training status). Rest 45 seconds between each set. Keep safety and proper form in mind as you slowly increase the weight lifted or the number of sets. Though novices often start out using weight machines, it's beneficial to progress to using free weights also.

- Give your muscles a day to recuperate between strengthening sessions. If you want to do resistance training daily, do a "split routine"—above the waist one day and below the waist the next.

- Do not hold your breath. Think "ee" or exhale on exertion.

- By making slow and controlled movements, you help to isolate the muscle groups you're working instead of using the momentum or swing of your body. Lift and return the weight to the slow count of 5.

- Carry your water bottle and hydrate between routines.

- Stay mindful as you focus on the muscle you are contracting and relaxing. This will improve the quality of your workout and make it more meditative.

- Try a resistance-training or body-sculpting class to add variety, fun, and skilled instruction to your workout.

- Home resistance-training programs are also available in books such as *Strong Women Stay Slim* by Dr. Miriam Nelson and *Strength Training Past 50* by Dr. Wayne L. Westcott and Dr. Thomas R. Baechle, and in exercise videos featured in Collage Video Catalogue (1-800-433-6769) (see Appendix C for other resources). Consult these books and videos regularly to learn new routines and challenge your muscles in new ways.

If you decide that using free weights, resistance bands, or multipurpose weight machines at home best fits your schedule, check out stores in your area that sell exercise equipment. Some equipment vendors will send out a free personal trainer with new equipment purchases. If you decide to join a fitness club to take advantage of the many weight machines available, see if personal trainers are available to help you develop a safe program. Many clubs also offer free orientations to the weight room and one free hour with a personal trainer upon joining. Commit to joining a health club, as it increases the likelihood that you will get hooked on exercise.

Success Boosters

A better understanding of exercise basics, such as stretching, aerobics, and resistance training, helps you to make smarter program choices. You also understand how to use the FITTE principle as your guide. And marking your progress is easy with the help of record keeping or a pedometer. Check your progress with these questions:

	Yes	No
■ Do I understand the importance of stretching?	___	___
■ Am I doing SDLs (stretches of daily living)?	___	___
■ Am I stretching before *and* after my planned exercise?	___	___
■ Am I using the FITTE principle to guide my exercise choices?	___	___
■ Am I marking my progress with a pedometer or a FITTE activity record?	___	___
■ Have I started a resistance-training program?	___	___
■ Am I getting the proper nutrition and hydration before, during, and after exercise?	___	___

All-or-Nothing Doer

Weight Busters
Adopt a Moderate Mind-Set

"When I'm on and focused, there's no stopping me. I stay committed twenty-four hours of the day until the job is done. And when I'm finished, I'm either onto the next deadline or it's total downtime." This scenario is fairly typical of my goal-oriented all-or-nothing doer patients who are either "on" or they're "off"—a personality trait they apply to all activities in their lives. Whether it's negotiating a business transaction, doing volunteer work, or tackling a home project, they typically give 100 percent until it's done. And the word "moderation" is a foreign one since this "on-and-off" strategy works for them most of the time. But they soon discover that it's a formula for disaster when it comes to exercise and weight control. Many all-or-nothing doers are weekend warriors exercising to the max, but come Monday morning they're sore, injured, or exhausted, leading to a week of recovery and inactivity. Up and down, on and off. Because weight management is a long-term, often lifelong, project without specific deadlines, adopting a moderate mind-set is my first prescription for you.

As an all-or-nothing doer, you probably feel that unless you can do your full workout, such as running for 30 minutes or biking for 45 minutes, it's not worth doing anything at all. First and foremost, you need to give yourself permission to do less.

> ⇒ *Nibble on This* ⇐
>
> Doing moderate workouts consistently is better than doing intense workouts inconsistently.

Studies show that you get health and psychological benefits from engaging in short bouts of activity. They add up, over the course of a day or even over several weeks. It's okay to run for only 15 minutes or bike for 20 minutes if that's all the time you have. That's because little bits of physical activity can go a long way to enhance mental alertness, improve sense of well-being, decrease depression, and even lengthen your life span. Some activity is always better than none. This sounds intuitive and rational but probably hard for you to accept since it's not your disposition. But I suggest you give this strategy a try. Once you appreciate how different exercise is from your other work projects (with actual start and stop dates), you'll make a conscious effort to dial back your extreme workouts. So if you can't run for 30 minutes before dinner, you know that walking for 10 minutes in the morning and at lunchtime is just fine—and much better than doing nothing at all.

Get Real

Setting realistic goals will help you to achieve the balance in your life that may be missing. On the days that you will not be able to get to the health club, make a point to increase your activities of daily living or ADLs. Whether it's walking your dog longer in the mornings and evenings, walking while waiting for an appointment, taking a walking break instead of a coffee break, or riding your bicycle to the drugstore, all activity counts and adds up to burning more calories. Wearing a pedometer on your belt is a great way to "get credit" for these extra motions throughout the day. No, these ADLs may not directly replace a 30-minute, high-intensity workout in the gym, but they are realistic and achievable on the days that you cannot enjoy a higher-level workout. Some patients also find that purchasing home exercise equipment gives them more options for moderating their exercise routines. So a half-hour evening walk on a home treadmill while watching a favorite television show gives the all-or-nothing doers other options—and convenient ones, at that.

> ⮑ *Nibble on This* ⬅
> When you have more activity options, being active doesn't have to be optional.

Understand Triggers

Although the first two strategies are extremely helpful in breaking your on-and-off exercise pattern roller coaster and initiating a new course, a longer-term strategy is to ask yourself what triggers the "on" cycle to exercise and, equally important, what triggers the "off" cycle. Once you understand these stop and start signals, you will be closer to taking back control of this cyclic behavior. Some patients say that time pressures are their biggest obstacle to regular exercise, but for others it's an acute injury or simply a change in mood. Take Ken, who gave it his all at the gym where he spent 2 hours combining aerobics and weight training, 5 times a week. But during Ken's "off" weeks, you would be lucky to see him even take the stairs one flight up. During treatment, Ken was able to moderate his workout routines, but self-reflection didn't come as easily. I helped Ken to realize that it was his wavering mood that changed his motivation. When he was in a good mood, he felt energetic, productive, and lively. In contrast, bad moods were associated with fatigue, low ambition, and poor concentration. This revelation led Ken to talk to a psychologist, who after several visits helped him better understand the emotional triggers that caused his mood swings. Once Ken learned how to take better control of these emotional triggers, he was also able to conquer his mood swings and cyclic exercise behaviors.

I use Ken's story to illustrate that every one of my all-or-nothing doer patients has his or her own personal triggers for starting and stopping exercise. Think about yourself. What prompts you to exercise? Is it just for weight loss or to combat a recent threat to your health, or are you also enjoying the benefits that exercise brings to your body and mind? And what are your triggers for stopping exercise? If injuries prevent you from exercising, you're probably doing too much without the proper warm-up and cooldown or you're progressing too quickly—more than 5–10 percent a week. Moderate your exercise routine and commit to doing pre- and postexercise stretches. Get a stretching book or video from the library with pictures and specific instructions on preventing exercise-related injuries. (*Stretching* by Bob Anderson is a good choice.) Add resistance training to your routine to make your muscles stronger and less prone to injury. Consult with a personal trainer who can teach you proper form and observe your technique in just a few sessions.

If a time problem is causing you to stop exercising, consider looking hour by hour over your daily schedule so you can prioritize fitness back into your routine. Many of my time-pressured patients find that getting up early to exercise is their only way to fit it in. Ask for help from family members or start delegating more at work. If stress is a factor, check out Chapter 5 for energizing and healthy ways to destress. And if the cost of your exercise routine is getting too high, consider cheaper ways to stay active and healthy by engaging in fitness walking or by using exercise videos at home (call Collage Video at 1-800-433-6769 for a free catalog).

Enjoy Building Skills

Once you better understand and take control over your start and stop exercise triggers, it's time to step it up a notch by taking on new exercise challenges and learning new skills. Your options are endless and range from tennis, raquetball, and spinning classes to swimming, hiking, ice skating, or snowshoeing. Personal interests usually dictate my patients' choices—along with the opportunities available where they live or work. One patient signed up for a weekly tennis class at a local park district while another joined a speed-walking group near her office. Still another patient joined a community fitness center with classes in yoga, dance aerobics, and fit ball strength training—activities that all piqued her interest.

It's time now for you to investigate your options, that is, the programs and classes offered in your community or near your workplace. Consider making this a social experience by engaging the support of an interested friend or family member. Or log on to an Internet weight loss chat group to see the types of activities other dieters enjoy doing. As you scrutinize your options, pick activities that challenge your body and sound fun. And remember that building new skills is a healthy way to feed your goal-oriented personality—with the added bonus of keeping you active.

> ⋙ *Nibble on This* ⋘
> Instead of changing your goal-oriented personality, try changing your goals.

Success Boosters

As you give yourself permission to do less, you're able to set more realistic goals that include moderating your extreme workouts. And trying to understand and overcome your exercise stop triggers has helped you to put a greater sense of balance back into your life. Monitor your progress with these questions:

	Yes	No
■ Have I adopted the mind-set that any activity is better than no activity?	___	___
■ Are my activity goals more realistic and achievable?	___	___
■ Do I better understand my exercise stop and start triggers?	___	___
■ Am I able to counteract my reasons for stopping to exercise?	___	___
■ Am I channeling my goal-oriented personality toward healthier pursuits: taking an exercise class and building new skills?	___	___

Set-Routine Repeater

Weight Busters
Change the Pace

Routine brings comfort, familiarity, and predictability into all of our lives. Yet for the set-routine repeater, doing the same thing over and over again may be just the reason you can't lose weight. Take Victoria, a 44-year-old woman who came in frustrated about her weight being at a standstill, despite doing a treadmill walking program 3 mornings a week. Victoria's 2.8-mph "stroll" was not challenging enough for her body, causing her to change the pace of her workout.

> ⇒ *Nibble on This* ⇐
>
> Using the same groups of muscles to perform the same aerobic activities makes your body efficient in performing the same work. More efficiency means you burn fewer calories.

The first three letters (*F*requency, *I*ntensity, and *T*ime) of the FITTE principle helped Victoria as they will guide you. If you are not working out at the right intensity (with a perceived exertion of a 6 or 7), then I first recommend that you increase your walking speed. Though increasing to a 1 or 2 percent incline is another option, I don't recommend this if you have knee or back problems. Next, I use the F (frequency) and T (time) of the FITTE principle to show how you can safely progress your workout even further using the 10 percent rule. For example, Victoria figured out that her current 40-minute, 3-times-a-week workout needed to increase by 12 minutes (10 percent of her total 120-minute weekly workout time). She decided that the easiest way to do this was to add 4 minutes to each day's workout. Another option would have been to increase her workout days to 4 and decrease the time of each workout to 33 minutes.

Let these examples guide you as you safely change the pace of your exercise routine.

Surprise Your Body

Whereas the first strategy gave you ideas on how to burn more calories doing the same workout routine, getting more fit and feeling more energetic (and even decreasing the occasional boredom you may feel from being a set routine repeater) requires that you vary your routine. That means stepping outside of your comfort zone—which may be always walking on the treadmill, or riding a stationary bike, or doing the same low-impact aerobic exercise video—and trying something new. And remember that as you lose weight, you'll be able to try new activities you were previously unable to do.

Surprise your muscles with new activities and surprise yourself by adding fun and enjoyment to your routine. Taking an exercise class of any kind is a great strategy for set-routine repeaters to try because an instructor motivates you to do more than you would do alone. Even if you're not a "class person," classes may be just what you need to stimulate your mind and body toward greater fitness and weight loss. You'll never know what you're capable of doing until you try. Take Jenna, who in her fifties started ice skating again after losing 20 pounds (15 years after hanging up her last pair of skates), which truly surprised her, her muscles—and her kids. Decide to vary the intensity and type of your workout routines. This table outlines activities ranging from light to vigorous.

Activities by Intensity

Light Activities	Moderate Activities	Hard/Vigorous Activities
Walking slowly (strolling)	Walking briskly	Walking vigorously or briskly uphill; running
Cycling, mild effort	Cycling, moderate effort	Cycling, fast or racing; spinning classes
Billiards	Table tennis, badminton, volleyball	Racquetball; competitive badminton or soccer
Golf, using power cart	Golf, pulling cart or carrying clubs	
Swimming, slow treading	Swimming, moderate effort	Swimming, crawl
Bowling	Tennis, doubles	Tennis, singles
Shuffleboard	Ice skating	Hiking and climbing
Boating, power	Rowing, canoeing, kayaking leisurely	Rowing, canoeing, kayaking rapidly
Playing musical instrument	Aerobic dancing; step aerobics; dance lessons	Cross-country skiing or snowshoeing; downhill skiing
Conditioning exercises: light stretching; yoga; Pilates (beginner); fit ball class	Conditioning exercises: power yoga; Pilates (intermediate or advanced)	Conditioning exercises: StairMaster or elliptical trainer; kick boxing; skipping rope
Fishing, sitting	Fishing, standing and casting	Fishing in stream
Horseshoe pitching	Horseback riding, walking, and trotting	Horseback riding, galloping
Weight training, body sculpting class	Circuit weight training	Backpacking
Source: Adapted from Russell Pate et al., *Physical Activity and Public Health*.		

Make a commitment to try one new activity each month and you'll be well on your way to breaking out of your routine.

Don't Resist Resistance

Many people who are used to doing aerobic exercise routines and sticking to them have yet to start a resistance-training program of any kind. This especially applies to postmenopausal women who are commonly frustrated that their weight has been climbing despite doing aerobics regularly. Previously convinced that her body did not work, Karen became a true believer in resistance training when she saw her dress size drop and her clothes fit better.

> ➣ *Nibble on This* ➢
>
> "You can regain approximately two decades' worth of age-associated losses in strength and muscle mass within about two months of resistance strength training."
>
> —HURLEY AND ROTH, *SPORTS MED*

Health experts agree that if you're doing only aerobics for weight loss, you're missing the boat, since strength training counteracts the decrease in muscle mass and metabolism accompanied by age—thus boosting weight loss. Ironically, the first thing I recommend you do when starting weight training is develop a set routine using free weights, resistance bands, circuit machines, or a combination. But just like aerobic exercise, if you stay at the same resistance (weight) for weeks on end, you will no longer be challenging your muscles. The key is to start out with proper instruction that can be provided by a personal trainer, exercise instructor, book, or video (see resistance training basics on page 106). And then with safety in mind, keep advancing your game.

You can keep challenging your muscles in many ways: by increasing the weight lifted, the number of repetitions, the number of sets, the type of exercise, or the speed (the slower the speed, the greater the resistance). Some patients progress to free weights instead of machines, which is harder as it requires them to stabilize their own body during lifting. Lifting while doing lunges or using a stability ball requires more work, as each adds instability to your movements. My patients quickly learn that if they want to increase their metabolism round the clock—24 hours a day—building lean muscle through resistance training is needed.

> ➣ *Nibble on This* ➢
>
> "A Tufts University study shows that women who diet and do strength training lose 44 percent more fat than the ones who diet only."
>
> —DR. MIRIAM E. NELSON WITH SARAH WERNICK, *STRONG WOMEN STAY SLIM*

Swim Against the Stream

Just as you are a set-routine repeater in your exercise, you may also be a routine repeater in your activities of daily living. Do you park in the same space every day at work, always take the elevator up or down one flight, or always drive one block to mail a letter? Swimming against the stream means doing it differently. When everyone else is standing on the escalator, you walk up. When your work colleagues are waiting for the elevator, you take the stairs down. Instead of giving your car to the valet, park it yourself. All these ADLs burn extra calories and will help you progress in your weight loss journey.

Success Boosters

You now have many ways to change the pace of your exercise routine. And along with choosing different types of activities (including resistance training), you're able to build muscle while boosting your weight loss—and enjoyment. Check your progress with these questions:

	Yes	No
■ Am I changing the frequency, intensity, and/or time of my exercise routine?	____	____
■ Am I trying new (and more vigorous) activities?	____	____
■ Am I enjoying exercise more?	____	____
■ Have I begun a resistance-training program?	____	____
■ Am I safely progressing my resistance-training program?	____	____
■ Am I increasing my ADLs?	____	____

Aches-and-Pains Sufferer

Weight Busters
Set Healthy Boundaries

Whether you have aches and pains in your joints, a sore foot, a bad back, a chest pain you're concerned about, or a health problem such as diabetes or high blood pressure, all aches-and-pains sufferers need medical clearance before embarking on an exercise program. The goal is to find exercises that are safe, sound, and effective for your particular condition. Before starting to exercise, I recommend that you consult with your personal physician about the following areas:

- Are any outside referrals necessary? Should you see a cardiologist for a stress test; a physical therapist for evaluation and treatment of neck, shoulder, arm, back, leg, knee, or hip problems; a podiatrist or orthopedic surgeon for evaluation and treatment of foot problems?
- Are there any types of stretches or exercises recommended for your condition? Will standing calf stretch, non-weight-bearing exercises, water exercise, recumbent bike, and/or chair exercises help you?
- Should any types of stretches or exercises specifically be avoided? Will lying hamstring stretch, jogging, and/or kick boxing harm you?
- Are there any precautions about exercising safely? Don't exercise in heat or humidity; don't twist or jump; be sure to warm up and cool down; if you experience dizziness, shortness of breath, or chest pain, stop and get help, use ice on aching joints before and after workouts if needed.

Consulting first with your physician will increase your chances of developing a safe and comfortable program—and one you will continue for life. For example, a podiatrist referral enabled one patient to resume a pain-free walking program, once she had the right orthotics in her walking shoes. A physical therapy referral gave another patient the daily exercise stretches that decreased his low back pain, increased his flexibility, and enabled him to get back to exercising without fear of injury.

If you don't already have a doctor or don't know if you have a problem that needs further evaluation before exercising, the following Physical Activity Readiness Questionnaire will guide you.

You may also be wondering whether you need a cardiac stress test before you start an exercise program. If you are a man under 45 or a woman under 55, have no symptoms or health concerns and no known medical problems such as high blood pressure, elevated blood cholesterol, diabetes, cigarette smoking, or early family history of heart disease, then you are categorized as low risk and a cardiac stress test is not necessary. On the other hand, if you do not meet the criteria I just listed, then you *may* need further evaluation, particularly if you plan to participate in moderately vigorous exercise. Once again, this is a conversation to have with your physician.

Physical Activity Readiness
Questionnaire - PAR-Q
(revised 1994)

PAR - Q & YOU

(A Questionnaire for People Aged 15 to 69)

Regular physical activity is fun and healthy, and increasingly more people are starting to become more active every day. Being more active is very safe for most people. However, some people should check with their doctor before they start becoming much more physically active.

If you are planning to become much more physically active than you are now, start by answering the seven questions in the box below. If you are between the ages of 15 and 69, the PAR-Q will tell you if you should check with your doctor before you start. If you are over 69 years of age, and you are not used to being very active, check with your doctor.

Common sense is your best guide when you answer these questions. Please read the questions carefully and answer each one honestly: check YES or NO.

YES	NO		
☐	☐	1.	Has your doctor ever said that you have a heart condition <u>and</u> that you should only do physical activity recommended by a doctor?
☐	☐	2.	Do you feel pain in your chest when you do physical activity?
☐	☐	3.	In the past month, have you had chest pain when you were not doing physical activity?
☐	☐	4.	Do you lose your balance because of dizziness or do you ever lose consciousness?
☐	☐	5.	Do you have a bone or joint problem that could be made worse by a change in your physical activity?
☐	☐	6.	Is your doctor currently prescribing drugs (for example, water pills) for your blood pressure or heart condition?
☐	☐	7.	Do you know of <u>any other reason</u> why you should not do physical activity?

If

you

answered

YES to one or more questions

Talk with your doctor by phone or in person BEFORE you start becoming much more physically active or BEFORE you have a fitness appraisal. Tell your doctor about the PAR-Q and which questions you answered YES.

- You may be able to do any activity you want — as long as you start slowly and build up gradually. Or, you may need to restrict your activities to those which are safe for you. Talk with your doctor about the kinds of activities you wish to participate in and follow his/her advice.
- Find out which community programs are safe and helpful for you.

NO to all questions

If you answered NO honestly to <u>all</u> PAR-Q questions, you can be reasonably sure that you can:

- start becoming much more physically active — begin slowly and build up gradually. This is the safest and easiest way to go.
- take part in a fitness appraisal — this is an excellent way to determine your basic fitness so that you can plan the best way for you to live actively.

DELAY BECOMING MUCH MORE ACTIVE:

- if you are not feeling well because of a temporary illness such as a cold or a fever — wait until you feel better; or
- if you are or may be pregnant — talk to your doctor before you start becoming more active.

Please note: If your health changes so that you then answer YES to any of the above questions, tell your fitness or health professional. Ask whether you should change your physical activity plan.

<u>Informed Use of the PAR-Q</u>: The Canadian Society for Exercise Physiology, Health Canada, and their agents assume no liability for persons who undertake physical activity, and if in doubt after completing this questionnaire, consult your doctor prior to physical activity.

Reprinted with permission from the 1994 revised version of the Physical Activity Readiness Questionnaire (PAR-Q and YOU). PAR-Q and YOU is a copyrighted, pre-excercise screen owned by the Canadian Society for Excercise Physiology.

Make It Short and Sweet

Despite your functional limitations, I recommend that you start with what you can do and build from there. Think small—add the little things you can do to build activity into your daily life: Walk to mail a letter, carry laundry loads up a flight of stairs, or walk to a neighbor's house to chat instead of E-mailing. Even a simple activity like taking your dog to a dog park or walking your child to and from school can keep you active and functioning at your best. These accumulated activities are a wonderful way to get in exercise without the fear of hurting yourself. You always remain in control of how much and what you are doing. But stay away from activities that can aggravate your condition (such as walking downstairs if you have knee problems). I recommend that you do the stretches of daily living, or SDLs, on page 101 regularly to stay as flexible as possible, again tailoring your program to your particular condition. And remember: Don't bounce, over-stretch, or stretch to the point of pain.

Small changes do make a big difference in both your sense of well-being and your weight. The benefits of physical activity can still be acquired by accumulating spurts of aerobic activity throughout the day—instead of all at once.

Go Alternative

Since many aches-and-pains sufferers may have difficulty either jumping straight into aerobics or advancing their aerobic routines, alternative activities like yoga, chair aerobics, tai chi, aquasize, or a fit ball muscle-strengthening class may be just the ticket. The Eastern practices of yoga and tai chi combine various stretches, poses, and movements to relax and challenge your body in new ways. And each motion can be executed to the level and degree of your own comfort and ability. Many yoga positions can be adapted to sitting if you have difficulty standing or lying for long periods of time. The cheapest entryway into yoga or tai chi is to purchase a videotape and follow along in your own home. However, to get the full benefit, consider taking a class.

Aquasize is a great option if you have arthritis. And those of you with bad backs may benefit from taking a fit ball class where you maintain your posture, increase your flexibility, and strengthen your core muscles using the stability ball. If you fear injuring yourself in an exercise class, the stability ball is a therapeutic tool that helps to support your lower back while you strengthen your abdominal muscles. Another side benefit to taking alternative-type activity classes is that they encourage you to focus on how keeping active reduces pain and stiffness and increases relaxation and flexibility. Exercisers even report having improved sleep, more energy, and better mood. And best of all these are fun classes for people of all ages. So check your local papers or even the Internet for classes in or around your neighborhood.

With a history of chronic knee pain, Linda found help through a combination of tai chi, aquasize, and a quadriceps strength-training program. Because Linda had a history of multiple knee injuries, her primary exercise goal was to not get hurt again. These alternative therapies helped Linda to succeed as her pain level decreased while her daily functioning, energy level, and mood all improved.

> ⧼ *Nibble on This* ⧽
>
> "Longevity is the maximum return on your exercise investment."
>
> —PEGGY MITCHELL, EXERCISE PHYSIOLOGIST, NORTHWESTERN MEMORIAL HOSPITAL WELLNESS INSTITUTE

Seek Supervision

To continue advancing your exercise program safely and effectively, chances are you will need to seek supervision for further instruction and monitoring. Proper and safe exercises are an absolute must to avoid any injury to your joints and muscles. Several of my patients have had their exercise program brought to an abrupt halt after injuring themselves on unfamiliar machines. My recommendation is that you be evaluated by an exercise professional, either at a health club or at a hospital wellness facility or cardiac rehab program. Those who join supervised programs feel more comfortable exercising aerobically, especially with the strong injury prevention focus on proper warm-ups and cooldowns.

Resistance training also decreases your pain and stiffness while increasing your metabolism and boosting weight loss. Safety precautions to follow include having a professional adapt a program to your specific injury or condition, being observed to ensure proper technique, and progressing your program slowly.

> ⧼ *Nibble on This* ⧽
>
> Stronger muscles are less injuryprone.

> ### ➣ *Nibble on This* ➢
> Respect the exercise time you schedule on your calendar as if it was your biggest client or closest friend. Honor appointments with yourself and don't break them.

If you have trouble honoring these appointments, enlisting the support of a friend or an exercise trainer, or even signing up for a class can help. Some external accountability may be all you need to follow through.

Multi-task Your Exercise

Multitasking, which means doing more than one activity or job at a time, is familiar to most of us who need to fit many things into our hectic lives. Common examples are having a business meeting over lunch or making work-related calls during the home commute. You can apply this same strategy to exercise by doing one or more of the following:

- Combine exercises such as aerobics or weight training with a favorite TV or radio show or book on tape—which helps the time go by quickly. Some individuals have also mastered the ability to read and exercise at the same time, but this is much more difficult and may actually hinder achieving a higher-intensity workout.
- Connect socially while exercising by doing fitness walks with friends, family members, or even work colleagues. Or sign up for a physically active class (dancing, aerobics, spinning, tennis, yoga) either with a friend or as an opportunity to meet new people.
- Exercise alone, using the time while walking, running, or cycling to solve work projects, resolve family problems, or clear your mind of the day's stresses.

Think about ways you can multitask your exercise, which can energize you and make you more productive both at work and at home.

Ask for Help

This strategy helps clear the way for a longer-term solution for fitting exercise into your life. Take a careful look at your "portfolio of responsibilities" and decide which ones you can delegate to others—both at work and at home. By shifting some of your work responsibilities to others, you allow them to grow and assume a higher level of accountability. The same can be said at home. Asking your children to take on more responsibility, such as making their own lunches, cleaning their rooms, or helping with the dishes, helps them mature. Your spouse or significant other also has a role to play in lightening your load—you just need to ask for help. By clearing your portfolio, you will be making more precious time for yourself: time for self-care and time to exercise.

Success Boosters

Since increasing ADLs takes the least time commitment on your part, this has become your number-one priority. And wearing a pedometer keeps you motivated as you track your progress. You're not only making weekly appointments with yourself, you're also actually keeping them. You multitask your exercise whenever possible and you're trying to delegate more at home and work. Check your progress with these questions:

	Yes	No
Am I increasing my ADLs?	____	____
Am I wearing a pedometer to track my progress?	____	____
Have I gone hour by hour over my daily calendar to find the time I need to exercise?	____	____
Am I prioritizing my health higher up on my to-do list?	____	____
Am I multitasking my exercise whenever possible?	____	____
Am I asking for help so that time is on my side?	____	____

Feeling Your Feelings

Now that you've added exercise to your routine, it's time to look at the feelings and situations that have derailed your good efforts in the past. The next chapter will help you improve your coping skills while better understanding and controlling your thoughts, feelings, and emotions.

Chapter 5

Shaping Your Coping Personality

I f stress can make you fat, as some researchers say, does that mean that coping better can make you thinner? Over the years, I noticed that those who improve their coping skills are more motivated to stick with the program and so sustain more weight loss. For many, learning better coping strategies is the missing piece to their weight loss puzzle. In this chapter, you will learn coping strategies that promise to improve your mood, increase your confidence, release tension, and strengthen the mental focus you need to lose weight. All you have to do to get started is pick one of your coping patterns.

Emotional Stuffer

Weight Busters
Inventory Food and Mood

For emotional stuffers, eating provides love, comfort, solace, and relief in response to emotional triggers such as anxiety, loneliness, stress, and depression. Using the ABC behavior chain, my patients "get to the heart" of their emotional eating. In this behavior chain, A is for the antecedents or what triggered the eating, B is for the behavior of eating or what you ate, and C is for the consequences or how you felt after eating.

> ⤜ *Nibble on This* ⤛
> The therapeutic power of a behavior chain is that it allows you both to under-
> stand and break habits that seem unbreakable.

Using the sample table below, draw three ABC columns on a sheet of paper or in a notebook. It's extremely important that you do this exercise on paper, as recording your thoughts will clarify links and triggers that initially appear unrelated. Take a few days (at least one weekday and one weekend day) to log any emotion-related eating. If you know that you're an emotional eater, but your diary doesn't demonstrate this, you may need to keep your diary longer until this pattern becomes apparent. The following is an example of what your entries may look like.

Sample ABC Food/Mood Behavior Chain Diary

Antecedents (emotional triggers that occur before eating)	Behavior (eating)	Consequences (feelings and attitudes that follow eating)
Home alone on Saturday night; feeling lonely	Ate 2 large bowls of ice cream.	Mood momentarily improved but then felt guilty and fat.
Disagreement with coworker; feeling anxious and frustrated	Grabbed candy bar and Coke from vending room at work.	Felt soothed at first. Able to get back to work as long as I avoided colleague. Then felt too jumpy from the caffeine and sugar.

If you haven't given a lot of thought to your emotional eating triggers, this self-revealing exercise may be hard for you. To make it easier, I developed a list of questions. Find a quiet place where you can think about and answer them as honestly as possible.

- How much of my planned or unplanned eating is emotional or stress related (for example, percent of time, number of snacks)?
- What are the most problematic situations or times that trigger emotional eating?
- How else do I cope with stress or my emotions?

As the answers to these questions raise your self-awareness, you will be better able to uncover your ABC food/mood behavior chain. Give yourself whatever time you need to accurately pinpoint your trigger emotions.

> ⇒ *Nibble on This* ⇐
>
> "Feelings are messages that tell you what you need."
>
> —Dr. Cindy Levin, psychologist, Northwestern Memorial Hospital Wellness Institute

Acknowledge Your Feelings

Once you start tracking your emotional triggers, you can begin to seriously acknowledge them. Instead of stuffing your emotions with food, you learn to interpret these feelings and meet your needs healthfully.

A higher level of emotional awareness is your goal—where you think about and experience your emotions—a strategy made easier with practice and journal writing.

To help you figure out your emotional eating triggers, I recommend that you add a forth column to your ABC diary titled "thoughts and reflections," so you can document your interpretations, which will help you to troubleshoot future situations. If you have an aversion to journaling, discuss your triggers with someone you trust. You'll know you're making progress once you're able to identify your emotional triggers—even before you reach for some food.

> ⇒ *Nibble on This* ⇐
>
> The healing process begins once you allow yourself to feel, experience, and better understand the emotions that cause you to eat.

Nurture Emotions Without Food

Over the years, eating has provided you a short-term fix for your different emotions as it seemed to soothe the soul when you were lonely or stressed, and to comfort you when you were depressed. As the emotional eating led to weight gain, however, these emotions were exacerbated and you came to see that food didn't really solve any problems. The strategy here is to problem-solve when you are *not* in the midst of the emotional trigger, preferably at a time when you can step back, re-create the situation, and think more clearly. Specifically, I want you to put into place an action plan for the next time the emotional trigger occurs. That means writing down in your notebook at least 4 alternative actions you can take for each emotional trigger. The following table shows the emotional eating action plan that Mary developed.

Mary's Emotional Eating Action Plan

Emotional Triggers	Loneliness	Stress at Work
Action Steps	1. Call a friend.	1. Do minirelaxation deep-breathing exercises.
	2. Log on to an Internet chat group.	2. Take a walking break outside (not to the vending machine).
	3. Write a letter to someone.	3. Talk it out.
	4. Visit a family member.	4. Journal my thoughts.

Now I want you to make your own list and keep it handy so you can use it the next time an emotional eating trigger strikes. With time, these new behaviors will become second nature and you will not have to keep referring to your lists. But be patient with yourself. You're still making progress even if you're able to identify your emotional eating trigger only while in the midst of eating. At whatever point you identify that emotion, you can stop eating and try to fill that need in other, more appropriate ways.

Strengthen Your Mind-Body Connection

Whereas the last strategy gave you short-term solutions to help you better deal with your emotional eating triggers, this strategy focuses on longer-term solutions. If your emotional eating is deeply rooted, you may benefit from trying some alternative practices that restore your ability to better deal with the stresses of everyday life. Through these activities, you learn how your body can strengthen your mind *and* how your mind can strengthen your body.

> ⇒ *Nibble on This* ⇐
>
> Mind-body activities decrease stress and improve your mood—naturally and without food.

Here are some mind-body activities that have helped emotional stuffers to cope with their feelings. Don't forget that a simple stretching and exercise program can be the quintessential mind-body activity.

Mind-Body Activities

Mindful Stretching and Exercise	Mindful Breathing/ Relaxation Exercises	Meditation	Yoga
Achieves calmness and energy through a stretching and exercise program that links your body movements with a dose of mindfulness.	Relaxes the mind and body through the power of breathwork or musclework.	Reduces tension and achieves calmness through quieting of your mind, which also calms your body.	"Yoga," which means unity or oneness, links the body to your mind and breath, while enhancing energy, calmness, and flexibility.
Massage	Imagery and Visualization	Pilates	Tai Chi
Soothes muscles and relieves tension of the mind and the body.	Enhances relaxation, reduces the stress response, and can even change behavior through using your senses and imagination.	Strengthens and tones core muscles while lengthening your body and relaxing your mind.	An ancient Chinese practice that uses relaxed, natural . movements to release tension and achieve balance and energy.

Try one or more of these activities. Check local papers or even the Internet for similar activities in or around your community. Or try relaxation tapes or videos at home. Find some time when you're not rushed and give these practices a try. You may discover that these activities really are "secrets" to making life easier. Once you start adding them to your life, their calming and energizing effects will motivate you to continue them.

Success Boosters

Now that you're more aware of your emotional eating triggers, you're able to acknowledge your feelings instead of stuffing them with food. And your emotional eating action plan (along with mind-body activities) gives you alternate and healthier ways to deal with your emotions. Check your progress with these questions:

	Yes	No
■ Am I using an ABC behavior chain to better understand my emotional eating?	____	____
■ Am I keeping a journal about my emotions?	____	____
■ Am I dealing with my emotions directly instead of stuffing them with food?	____	____
■ Have I developed an emotional eating action plan?	____	____
■ Have I identified mind-body activities I'd like to try?	____	____
■ Have mind-body activities helped me deal better with day-to-day stresses?	____	____

Low-Self-Esteem Sufferer

Weight Busters
Be Real About Body Image

Everyone has a self-image. For many people, it is closely tied to their occupation or their lifestyle. But for low-self-esteem sufferers, their self-image is closely tied to their body image or a distorted perception of what their body looks like to others. So the readings on their bathroom scale or the measurements around their waist and hips seem more important than what they do for a living, their intelligence, or their personal values. To break the vicious cycle of your distressing body image causing a poor self-image and low self-esteem, my first recommendation is to be more realistic about your body.

> ⤳ *Nibble on This* ⥆
>
> Just as you can't credit your appearance or body image for all your life successes, you also can't blame it for all your failures.

You can't keep putting your self-esteem on hold until you lose the weight—especially since losing weight doesn't ensure a positive body image—or even happiness, for that matter. This means that you need to work on accepting your body and learning to love and appreciate yourself now, not 40 pounds from now. In his book *What Do You See When You Look in the Mirror?* Dr. Thomas Cash, a pioneer in the psychology of physical appearance, discusses the importance of challenging traditional body image assumptions that cause distress. I will list two of them here to give you practice challenging the thoughts that can feed negative body image.

> ➤ *Nibble on This* ⇐
>
> "Negative body image has little to do with outward appearance; it's a state of mind."
>
> —DR. THOMAS CASH, *WHAT DO YOU SEE WHEN YOU LOOK IN THE MIRROR?*

I asked my patient Robin to journal her thoughts and try to challenge the following assumptions. Specifically, I asked her to figure out why these statements were *not* true. Dr. Cash says that this exercise helps you to "cultivate a new inner voice" that thinks about body image in a more realistic perspective.

1. By controlling my appearance, I can control my social and emotional life.
2. My appearance is responsible for much of what has happened to me in my life.

Robin's rebuttal of statement 1: "Losing all the weight and improving my appearance doesn't ensure that I would meet someone or that I would be happier. I remember when Judi lost so much weight, she became anorexic and was still miserable. Controlling her appearance sure didn't ensure her happiness."

Robin's rebuttal of statement 2: "When I think about it, my appearance really has nothing to do with how I've raised my children, or run my business—my two biggest accomplishments in life."

Now it's time for you to refute your body image assumptions. Write down what makes sense and what you would like to believe, and then take a few minutes daily to read them aloud. With time, you'll realize that you can control how you feel about your body—which will make you feel better about yourself.

> ⇒ *Nibble on This* ⇐
> "The more we like ourselves, the more easily we change and grow."
> —SUSAN KANO, *MAKE PEACE WITH FOOD*

Affirm Yourself

In many ways, low-self-esteem sufferers have been strangers to themselves. With such a strong focus on your negative characteristics, you probably have been unable to see or appreciate your positive qualities. That's sure to change once you understand that you *do* have the power to heal yourself—just by changing your thinking.

Think of people you care about and how you view them. Do you think about them or describe them in terms of their body parts or instead in terms of their personality traits and characteristics? Once you start treating yourself with the same dignity and respect as you treat others, your self-acceptance will grow. To counteract the excessive attention you give to your perceived physical weaknesses, think about your positive qualities and make a list of them. If this exercise is difficult for you to do alone, ask someone you trust to help you develop your list. Below is Beth's list.

- I have a good sense of humor.
- I'm a good listener.
- I have a strong religious faith.
- I'm a considerate person.
- I'm a nurturing parent of two children.
- I'm a loving spouse.
- I'm a kind daughter.
- I'm a trusted colleague at work.

- I'm artistic.
- My friends can always count on me.
- I'm a good third-grade teacher.
- I care a lot about my students.

Beth's self-affirmations above are all positive—quite different than the feelings of inadequacy voiced during her initial visit. Though Beth discussed her history of having low self-esteem (being told she was fat as a child), I reminded her that she was the adult in charge now of her feelings—and her self-esteem.

> ### ⇒ *Nibble on This* ⇐
> "Self-esteem is not a gift you can receive from someone else. It is generated from within."
> —NATHANIEL BRANDEN, *THE SIX PILLARS OF SELF-ESTEEM*

As with other low-self-esteem sufferers, I told Beth that if she wanted to move forward in this weight loss program, she needed to treat herself with more love and respect. Focusing on Beth's qualities redirected her energies positively toward her self-worth. Beth felt proud of the list she developed and even referred to it now and then whenever she doubted herself. Consider your list to be a symbol of self-awareness that will keep developing and improving, as your self-love deepens in this program.

Dismiss the Judging Committee

You're used to being lectured to—that is, by yourself, and you can be your own worst enemy, as evidenced by the frequent self-defeating thoughts that often replay in your mind like a broken record. Learn that these thoughts only worsen feelings of stress and negatively affect mood and behavior.

For many, this negative self-talk is so automatic that they have trouble hearing it. In fact, I often encourage them to slow down and quiet their minds long enough so they can hear their self-punishing thoughts. Eileen, for example, needed to sit in a quiet room alone for a while before her negative comments surfaced: "My hips are huge" and "I look like a fat slob." Once Eileen was able to bring these comments out into the open, I used a behavioral technique called cognitive restructuring so she could counteract these harsh messages. Instead of making automatic, critical judgments, Eileen learned to use factual words and phrases with specific information, not generalities.

Cognitive Restructuring

Automatic Negative Thinking	Restructured Positive Thinking
"My hips are huge."	"I have other clothes that better complement my body."
"I look like a fat slob."	"My weight is 210 pounds. I am dressed neatly but wish I could wear more stylish clothes."

Eileen also learned to use the STOP method of destressing (from the three-week plan) to change these thoughts from negative to positive: S—slow down, T—take a breath, O—observe objectively without attitude or emotion, P—plan a different response. But rather than restructure her thoughts so everything seemed perfect and rosy, the goal of this exercise was for her to become kinder toward and more understanding of herself. Sometimes Eileen also found that her sense of humor allowed her to step back and observe the situation as more of an outsider. She would catch her negative thought and then say, "I need to stop that evil Eileen. She never has anything nice to say." As these strategies helped Eileen's self-talk to become less distorted and more realistic, her mood and self-acceptance also improved.

Now it's time for you to think about any distorted thinking you have that keeps pounding away at your self-esteem. Take the time you need (just as Eileen did) just to think. As negative thoughts come to you, write them down. Once you have a list of recurring negative thoughts, use the following questions to restructure your thinking from negative to positive. Again, your goal is to treat yourself with the same dignity and respect with which you would treat a friend.

- What is the evidence that my thinking is true?
- Am I exaggerating the truth?
- Is there another, more rational and constructive, way to look at the situation?

Cognitive restructuring does take time, practice, and patience. But the rewards are great and well worth the effort. As you start treating yourself better, you'll also start feeling better. This will free your mind to think more clearly and make better day-to-day decisions that affect your weight—and your life.

Befriend Your Body

Just as a good relationship doesn't just happen and partners need to work on improving their relationship, a good body image doesn't just happen. This means that you need to work on improving your relationship with your body. How do you treat it and how does it treat you?

If you think that your body is the enemy, just the thought of befriending your body and strengthening your mind-body connection may be foreign to you.

Maria had thought that being fat meant she was a bad person. Through journaling and talking about her feelings, Maria worked on improving her inner sense of who she was. Taking a mindfulness class with a focus on relaxation exercises also helped Maria to carry out the healthier lifestyle behaviors that had previously eluded her. Within 5 months, Maria's hard work paid off, as her weight went from 326 to 252—a drop of 74 pounds. To put this strategy into action, I recommend that you begin by choosing one or more of the mind-body activities on page 129. Regular massages, though expensive, can be a wonderful way to nurture your body and mind. Try a yoga class that encourages mind-body flexibility and relaxation. Or take a regular meditation time in the morning or evening. And don't forget that the many types of physical exercise include other fun ways to strengthen your body image and raise your self-confidence.

The last way to befriend your body involves tuning in to the many sensual experiences that your body can enjoy, such as having sex; soaking in a Jacuzzi or hot tub; wearing sensual fabrics or perfume; rubbing scented lotion onto your body; getting a makeover; having a scalp massage; treating yourself to a manicure, pedicure, or facial; wearing comfortable, warm fabrics on a cold day; taking a relaxing shower or bubble bath, expressive dancing; or getting a new haircut.

> ⤐ *Nibble on This* ⤛
>
> "When you give your body what it really needs, including moderate exercise, healthful foods, sensual pleasures and relaxation, your body will respond by treating you better."
>
> —JUDITH RODIN, *BODY TRAPS*

As you treat your body better, your body image will improve, which in turn will increase your desire to treat your body better. It's a feedback loop that reinforces a stronger mind-body connection. If befriending your body is difficult because you avoid intimate relations or feel you don't deserve sensual pleasures, then you may need professional help (see Chapter 8).

Success Boosters

Now that you're able to think about your body image with a more realistic perspective, you realize that you are more than what you weigh. And you're trying to focus on your positive qualities, which you previously ignored. Cognitive restructuring and befriending your body are helping to improve your body image and your self-esteem. Check your progress with these questions:

	Yes	No
■ Am I trying to separate my weight from my self-esteem?	____	____
■ Am I trying to look at my body image in a more realistic light?	____	____
■ Am I refuting body image assumptions that cause distress?	____	____
■ Did I make a list of my positive qualities?	____	____
■ Do I refer to the list when needed?	____	____
■ Am I using cognitive restructuring or humor to change my negative self-talk?	____	____
■ Does the STOP method of destressing help me to better deal with my negative self-talk?	____	____

- Am I trying to improve my relationship with
  my body?   ____   ____
- Have mind-body activities, exercise, or sensual
  pleasures helped to improve my body image?   ____   ____

Persistent Procrastinator

Weight Busters
Probe Procrastination Trait

Though everyone procrastinates now and then, for the persistent procrastinator it's a habit or personality trait that regularly gets in the way of personal achievements. Interestingly enough, the first strategy is not one that
motivates you to start taking action. Instead, it's reflective in nature so you
can better understand the habit that keeps holding you back. Sit quietly and
observe your thinking as you review the following:

1. Pick one habit or target behavior (for example, eating healthier,
   exercising, destressing) that you keep consciously avoiding.
2. Write a list of the *benefits* of doing the chosen behavior, such as
   you will be a better role model for your children and will have
   more energy and feel better (from exercising).
3. Write a list of the *efforts* that will be needed to carry out the
   chosen behavior, such as the time needed away from work to
   exercise or the added expense of taking an exercise class.
4. Write a list of the *benefits* that result from *not* doing the behavior,
   such as you will not have to change anything and will be able to
   spend the same amount of time at work.

These thoughts and reasons are key to overcoming your procrastination
habit. Though the benefits of doing or not doing the behavior are usually
straightforward, the efforts needed to carry out the behavior often require
modifications in your daily routine. By finding the simplest ways to make
those modifications, change will begin to occur.

Try to identify other areas where you take risks and the character
strengths that help you to do so. Realizing that you can use these same
strengths to break the procrastination habit helps you to cope better with risk

taking. If you have trouble analyzing your procrastination habit on your own, try eliciting the support of someone you trust to assist you in problem-solving about ways to overcome any identified obstacles. And after you've had success with one targeted behavior, apply the same questions to a different behavior.

> ⤜ *Nibble on This* ⤛
>
> "It takes peace of mind and clarity to recognize and reorder meaningful, personal priorities."
>
> —SARAH BAN BREATHNACH, *SIMPLE ABUNDANCE*

Prompt Yourself

You've thought it through and have made a commitment to tackle a targeted behavior. Give yourself some extra help to ensure your success. The following are reminder prompts my persistent procrastinator patients place around the house to make taking action easier.

- preprinted grocery list with healthy options that you can circle week to week
- fresh fruit basket on counter
- notes to remind self to drink more water
- leaving water bottle out on counter
- healthy recipes to try
- stretching book and exercise mat in your bedroom
- gym clothes laid out the night before
- gym bag by the door
- scheduling workout dates with others
- placing workout equipment in sight
- using Palm Pilot for exercise reminders
- meditation tape next to the boom box
- eye pillow by your bed
- bubble bath next to the tub

- inspiring sayings on your message board
- candles by the dinner table

Consider these cues to be like secret love notes you've written and left around the house for a special loved one to find—yourself.

Make It Manageable

One thing that holds procrastinators back is thinking that weight loss requires a complete overhaul of their lifestyle. For nearly a decade of his life, Tom procrastinated about improving his eating and exercise habits until he discovered through my program how his "black-and-white thinking" stifled his best efforts. Tom was thrilled to learn that he didn't need to become a vegetarian or a competitive athlete to lose weight and get healthier. This adjustment in his thinking motivated Tom to make small changes in his lifestyle.

To keep you moving in the right direction, I recommend that you counter your procrastination reflex with a do-it-now attitude. Ask yourself, "What small thing can I do today to start achieving my goals?" And to decrease any overwhelmed feelings you may have about tackling your targeted behavior, break it up into manageable pieces and build it into your daily schedule. This takes just a few minutes of planning each day. For example, instead of deciding to exercise more, make a list of one or two things you can do to be more active each day—and then do them. Or instead of deciding that you will begin your diet tomorrow, say that today you will buy more fruits and vegetables at the grocery store, and tomorrow you will eat a fruit or vegetable with every meal or snack. Even if you pick just one small thing to do each day, you will be demonstrating your ability to take action and stop procrastinating.

Enjoy Small Successes

Many people often don't notice their small successes and don't use them to reinforce the process of change until they're pointed out to them. I encourage you to pay attention to yours, whatever they are. Whether you're buying more fruits and vegetables, not supersizing your fast-food meal, taking the stairs instead of the elevator, or using the STOP method of destressing, give yourself credit for this new behavior. It helps some of my patients to document their small successes daily in a journal. Others like to reward themselves regularly for carrying out their positive actions consistently. If you feel that journaling will help to reinforce your positive behaviors, then do so. If you find the thought of rewarding yourself to be motivating, then develop a list of healthy rewards you can choose from (do a fun activity with a friend, pamper yourself, rent a video, have a romantic night out with your mate, put money away for a special occasion). Going public with people you trust can also increase accountability and help you to stay on track.

Though small successes are great motivators, remember that this doesn't mean that small defeats should send you into a downward spiral—they're an expected part of the process. Learn from them. If you slip up and overeat at a meal, don't beat yourself up. Instead, think through how you can do better next time, and remember how far you've come.

> ⋟ *Nibble on This* ⋞
>
> "Success is the ability to constantly correct—like a thermostat."
>
> —Dr. Johanna Mytko, psychologist, Northwestern Memorial Hospital Wellness Institute

Success Boosters

Now that you've analyzed your procrastination habit, you understand yourself better and can problem-solve more effectively. For the behaviors you decide to carry out, you know that prompting yourself, making them manageable, and enjoying small successes all help you to stop procrastinating. Monitor your progress with these questions:

	Yes	No
■ Do I better understand my procrastination habit?	____	____
■ Did I devise a workable plan to overcome obstacles for each targeted behavior?	____	____
■ Do prompts make taking action easier?	____	____

- Am I breaking up the targeted behavior into
  manageable steps?   ____   ____
- Am I noticing my small successes?   ____   ____
- Am I journaling about or rewarding myself for
  my small successes?   ____   ____

Can't-Say-No Pleaser

Weight Busters
Understand the Disease to Please

Pleasers appear nice on the outside yet feel resentful on the inside—frequently saying yes to favors and added responsibilities when they really want to say no. But while you might be gaining points with your friends, relatives, or colleagues, you're losing valuable time that could have been devoted to uncovering and satisfying your own needs and desires. And in our fast-paced world where people never seem to have enough time or energy, this can negatively impact your mental and physical well-being. Once you better understand the disease to please, you're more willing to talk seriously about kicking the habit.

> ⋙ *Nibble on This* ⋘
> Sometimes you need to give yourself permission to say no.

The following table compares some typical feelings and reactions of a people pleaser versus a life passion pleaser. Instead of just wanting to give of their time and energy out of pure generosity, people pleasers act out of fear and the desire to avoid conflict. In fact, saying yes appears easier (at least, in the short run) than does saying no. But in the long run, those automatic yes responses do more harm than good as they eat up valuable time and energy for activities that may be totally out of line with your own goals and desires. So you end up without the time to do (or even think about) the things that have real meaning to you—your life passions.

People Pleaser vs. Life Passion Pleaser

	People Pleaser	Life Passion Pleaser
Response to a request for a favor or taking on more responsibilities	Gives automatic knee-jerk yes response without thinking	Knows time and energy are limited so gives serious thought to all requests before giving answer; says, "Let me think about it"
Motivator to saying yes	Seeks approval of others; hates confrontation or conflict	Is generous with her time if she knows it's something that's meaningful to her and consistent with her life passions
Feelings after saying yes to a request	Feels resentful	Feels fine
Feelings after saying no to a request	Feels selfish and guilty	Feels confident and assured
Most important approval source	Others	Herself

Pleasers need to learn that being selfish is quite different from purely caring for your own emotional and physical needs. In fact, investing in your health helps ensure you'll be around longer to take care of your loved ones. And self-care practices also show friends and family that you value yourself, which makes you a better role model. Seeking the approval of yourself instead of the approval of others is a challenge, but not an impossible one. As pleasers practice turning up the volume of their own voices and diminishing the volume of others', the results can actually be quite pleasing.

> ➤ *Nibble on This* ➤
>
> "You're not born a people-pleaser. People-pleasing is something you learn and can unlearn."
>
> —DR. HARRIET BRAIKER, *THE DISEASE TO PLEASE*

Envision Your Yeses

In *How to Say No Without Feeling Guilty*, Patti Breitman and Connie Hatch discuss how busyness can distract you from remembering the things in life that truly excite you. So before you gain the much-needed practice in learning how to say no, they suggest that you first envision your life yeses. The following questions will help you.

- What life passions drive you to say yes to things?
- Is there a correlation between your life passions and how you spend your time?
- If you had extra time, what activities would you want to fill it with that would give your life more meaning?
- What relationships would you want to nurture?

Let the table below help you to think through different options regarding your relationship, work, spiritual, and self-care life passions.

Life Passions Inventory

Relationship	Work	Spiritual	Self-Care
Find a true mate.	Seek a promotion.	Volunteer in the community.	Pursue a hobby.
Spend more time with family and friends.	Become self-employed.	Attend religious services.	Take a cooking class.
Adopt a baby.	Change careers.	Read inspiring books.	Attend a financial investment seminar.
Take a family vacation.	Work fewer hours.	Give to charitable causes.	Join a fitness center.
Get a dog.	Learn a new aspect of the business.	Work in religious school or choir.	Slow down and experience nature.

Though it's not unusual for people to do quick, mental life survey reviews now and then, few regularly write in a journal about their life passions. This recommended exercise can especially help pleasers change their focus from caring only about others' needs to also caring about their own. Note that I'm not recommending that you be self-centered, as your life passions inventory will encourage you to embrace the important people and causes in your life. Take the time you need to complete your own inventory. And remember that just as life changes, so do one's passions.

Say No Like a Pro

Up until now, saying no to others has probably conjured up feelings of fear. But now that you better understand your life passions, you can respond with more confidence and integrity. Here's a two-step process to strengthen your resolve:

1. Buy thinking time

    Buying thinking time is a crucial first step because it breaks your automatic yes response. When asked for a favor or request, common phrases that buy you thinking time are, "I need to check my calendar first," "Let me talk it over with my spouse," or "Let me think about it and I'll get back to you." These simple phrases give you the control to decide whether the request is in or out of line with your life passions inventory. If it is something meaningful to you and you have the time to do it, say yes. If it's not meaningful to you, say no.

2. Practice, but don't expect perfection

    Pleasers don't have a lot of experience dealing with the aftermath of saying no, which can result in others feeling disappointed or actually trying to change your mind. Since some situations will have better results than others, don't expect perfection as you practice saying no. Breitman and Hatch suggest that gaining practice by saying the "small no's" in life (to a telemarketer on the phone or to a clerk at a store) will increase your confidence to deal with the "bigger no's." So, too, making your responses short and to the point will avoid making you feel that every no requires an elaborate story. It doesn't. "No" is a complete sentence. As you start saying no more often to the things you don't want to do, you will be more available to the people and things you care about. Some people will still try to make you feel guilty, but your life will go on—with *your* guidance and approval, not theirs. Instead of always being the first one to call her friends when a problem arose, Rhonda had to give herself permission to put her own needs above those of her friends. Rhonda learned that she could still be a good friend without feeling responsible for the happiness of others.

> ➣ *Nibble on This* ➢
>
> "If you say no with your voice, you will no longer need to say it with your body weight."
>
> —GENEEN ROTH, *WHEN YOU EAT AT THE REFRIGERATOR, PULL UP A CHAIR*

Learn to Delegate

Since pleasers have a tendency to take on more than they can handle, delegating tasks to others helps to lighten their load—and build confidence in the process. Family and friends are not mind readers. It's healthy to teach people in your life that you have needs too. Family members have a responsibility to help you fulfill those needs. Confiding in them about your pleasing problem will help them to better understand you. Be specific when you ask for help: "I need you to pick up the cleaning on the way home from work so I have more time to prepare dinner" or "I need you to pick up the kids at soccer so I can attend my yoga class." It will ensure that you get the specific help you need.

Success Boosters

Now that you better understand the disease to please, you're making a conscious effort to say yes to the things that bring your life meaning. And as you learn to say no and delegate more, you're gaining extra time for yourself. Check your progress with these questions:

	Yes	No
■ Do I better understand the disease to please?	____	____
■ Did I complete my life passions inventory?	____	____
■ Is this list helping me choose when to say no or yes?	____	____
■ Am I buying time whenever I'm asked for a favor?	____	____
■ Am I practicing saying no without expecting perfection?	____	____
■ Am I trying to delegate more tasks than I used to?	____	____

Fast Pacer

Weight Busters
Notice Life Imbalances

By doing everything, fast pacers learn that something has to give—and it's often eating healthy, exercising, sleeping, or relaxing. In trying to control your frenetic pace of life, multitasking helps you pack more activities into your schedule. But it can also result in feelings of anxiety, stress, and lack of focus.

> ### ⮞ Nibble on This ⮜
> Working more and enjoying it less signals that your life is out of balance.

Becoming more aware of your life imbalances is an essential first step to taking back control and restoring a healthier balance. In their book *Living in Balance*, Dr. Joel and Michelle Levey suggest that one way to evaluate your life imbalances is by listing and then analyzing your life roles and identities. Complete a life roles inventory like the one below by thinking about and recording the various roles that comprise your identity. As you can see, this table builds on your previous life passions inventory. Different from the passions inventory that involves things you want to do in life, this inventory involves how you define yourself as a person. For each column, list as many roles (big or small) as you can think of, without being critical or scrutinizing them. Reflecting seriously about your life roles in the four areas of relationships, work, spiritual, and self-care will help you to better understand and then allocate how you spend your time.

Life Roles Inventory

Relationships	Work	Spiritual	Self-Care
▪ Husband	▪ Salesman	▪ Member of congregation	▪ Music lover
▪ Dad	▪ Business leader	▪ Spiritual person	▪ Golfer
▪ Son	▪ Computer buff	▪ Community member	▪ Sports fan
▪ Brother	▪ Program developer	▪ Fund-raiser	▪ Healthy person
▪ Friend	▪ Business association member	▪ Volunteer	▪ Avid reader

Take whatever time you need to think about and then answer the following questions about your inventory. Feel free to circle some responses as well.

■ How invested are you in each of the relationship, work, spiritual, and self-care areas?
■ Are you overextended in some areas?
■ Are other areas underdeveloped?
■ What areas are your greatest sources of stress?
■ If work, for example, is your greatest source of stress, how much time do you spend in other areas to balance that stress?
■ What areas are your greatest sources of joy?
■ If relationships are your greatest source of joy, how much time do you spend nurturing them?
■ Can you identify the areas of life that you want to develop more, along with the ones you want to cut back?

When Rick reflected on his inventory, he concluded that he needed to devote more time to his self-care roles to improve his health, which would then make him better able to fulfill his other life roles. Deep down Rick knew that his fast-paced lifestyle was leading him in the direction of developing one role that he didn't want—the sick role—if he didn't start to slow down and reprioritize.

Use Mindfulness to Self-Correct

Now that you have a better idea of the ways you want to use your time, the next step is to learn to appreciate and enjoy each and every role that you truly care about. This is called mindfulness. Many experts agree that mindfulness helps you to live the kind of purposeful and balanced life you desire. Mindfulness means slowing down, doing one activity at a time, and using all your senses (sight, sound, taste, touch, and smell) so that you fully experience the activity. Instead of being distracted and feeling stressed, mindfulness can help you to feel calmer as you maintain full awareness from moment to moment. This heightened sense of focus helps fast pacers to slow down and gain more enjoyment out of life as they rebalance their priorities.

The first step to changing your tendency toward being distracted or living mindlessly is to force yourself to pause in the course of your hectic day to break this habit, one way being through the practice of mindful breathing exercises.

Mindful Breathing Basics	
Purpose:	Mindful breathing is a relaxation skill where you become aware of tension in your body during inhalation and practice releasing tension during exhalation. Since breathing can be thought of as your link to the outside world, focusing on it allows your mind and body to become better harmonized with your surroundings.
Ways to do it:	As you slowly breathe in through your nose to the count of 4, relaxing your stomach allows it to rise (called diaphragmatic breathing). And as you slowly exhale through your mouth to the count of 4, your stomach falls. Repeat this process several times until you start to feel better. If you feel lightheaded or dizzy, however, resume normal breathing, as you may have been hyperventilating.
When to practice:	Whenever you feel stressed, overwhelmed, irritated, or distracted.

The Leveys suggest that another way to break your habit of mindlessness is to identify a routine (such as wearing your wristwatch on the same arm) and then change it (by wearing it on the opposite arm). Then whenever you catch yourself looking at the other wrist, you will be reminded to pause, take a calming breath, and break your routine by focusing your attention on the present moment.

> ➣ *Nibble on This* ➢
>
> "Living mindfully means more than just noticing things; it's that you're aware that you're noticing."
> —JOEL AND MICHELLE LEVEY, *LIVING IN BALANCE*

Your heightened sense of awareness helps you to better connect with others, feel more at ease with yourself, and better appreciate life's most basic pleasures. So you may eat, walk, and interact with more purpose and intention. Instead of seeing meals and working out as "just something to fit into your day," you may start seeing them as sacred times that honor your body and health. Rather than worrying about the past or the future, mindfulness reminds you to live in the present moment. It encourages you to make the most of events you can control.

Squeeze in Support

Mindful living helps fast pacers to rediscover the supportive people in their lives, those people whom they may have previously let slip by. Because fast pacers have type A personalities and typically handle complex tasks themselves (thinking they can do things better and faster than anyone else), they're used to getting the job done alone and without having to ask for help. In the process, however, you become overwhelmed and are unable to find time for good self-care. Seeking support in three different environments—home, work, and social—will help you balance your priorities.

Think about the following:

- What can you ask your loved ones at home to do to help you to handle stress better and find that extra time that you deserve (for example, give you some quiet time when you come home from work so you can wind down, respect your desire for a relaxing home atmosphere by not yelling or playing loud music, help out more with chores, allow you time away from home for exercise or for other self-care needs)?
- What really needs to be taken care of today?
- What can you delegate to coworkers to help decrease your workload?
- What can you simply stop doing?
- Think about the people in your life whom you enjoy spending time with versus the ones who drain your energy. Nurturing a supportive social network can be an excellent stress reducer.

Cheryl Richardson, author of *Take Time for Your Life*, suggests a different way to seek support: actually hire someone to help you. If you're unsure if you need this kind of help, she says to keep a list of tasks you do each day that someone else could easily do for you. Then by weighing the value of your time versus the cost of hired help, you can decide if this solution will work for you.

Revitalize Regularly

Though everyone needs to recharge his or her batteries now and then, this is especially important for fast pacers who normally tend to run on overdrive. Getting enough hours of restful sleep needs to be higher up on your to-do list.

> ### ⋙ Nibble on This ⋘
>
> "New research points to a possible connection between impaired sleep quality in men and hormonal changes that are associated with abdominal obesity."
>
> —DR. EVE VAN CAUTER, ET AL., *AGE-RELATED CHANGES IN SW SLEEP AND REM SLEEP AND RELATIONSHIP WITH GROWTH HORMONE AND CORTISOL LEVELS IN HEALTHY MEN*, JOURNAL OF THE AMERICAN MEDICAL ASSOCIATION

Certainly the mind-body activities on page 129 can help you to better manage stress during your waking hours, which in and of itself can foster better sleeping habits. These activities also give you other options for revitalizing regularly. I highlight relaxation exercises here because they are some of the easiest skills to learn and carry with you for life.

Relaxation Exercises

Purpose:	To quiet the mind and relax the body to achieve the relaxation response.
How to prepare:	Find a quiet room, loose clothing, and a comfortable position such as sitting in a chair or lying on the floor.
How to do it:	Once you're comfortable, close your eyes. As you focus on your breathing, relax your muscles starting with your head and face and moving down your neck, shoulders, arms, trunk, abdominals, legs, feet, and toes. Stay relaxed as you silently repeat a positive or neutral word ("peace," "love," "one") while slowly breathing in and then out. Continue breathing slowly and naturally for 10–20 minutes. If thoughts come to mind, silently repeat your chosen word and focus on your breath to help you dismiss them.
How you may feel afterward:	Most people experience relaxing and calming effects. Others feel refreshed, energized, and focused. Still some others may initially feel no different.
How often to do it:	If you practice it daily or even twice daily for a few weeks, you may notice great calming effects. If this is unrealistic for you, then do what works, such as starting it on the weekends only and then moving toward weekdays. A shorter version of these exercises can be used during times of high stress when you choose to do a shorter or minirelaxation session, for example in the middle of a hectic workday.

Some people find that relaxation exercises work better with the help of relaxation audiotapes (see Appendix C for information).

Aside from revitalizing regularly, fast pacers benefit from making small changes in their environment that help them to focus better and feel less distracted. In fact, they are usually surprised at how refreshing it can be to make the following simple changes:

At home: Clear clutter; create a special place where you can meditate or just unwind; place scented candles in bedroom, around bathtub, or near dining area.

At work: Clear clutter from desk; find quiet place where you can eat lunch without being disturbed; keep family pictures and plant on desk.

> ➤ *Nibble on This* ➤
>
> The physical clutter at home and work distracts and can cause psychological clutter in your mind.

Just as mind-body activities give fast pacers a much-needed break from their stressful lifestyle, clearing clutter revitalizes you as it clears the way for living a life of balance and intention.

Success Boosters

Now that you've noted your life imbalances, mindfulness is helping you to rebalance your priorities. And mindful breathing quickly refocuses you on the present moment. As you learn to ask others for help, you free up some time so you can revitalize yourself regularly. Check your progress with these questions:

	Yes	No
■ Did completing my life roles inventory help me to identify my life imbalances?	____	____
■ Is mindfulness helping me to bring my life back into better balance?	____	____
■ Does mindful breathing help me focus on the present moment?	____	____

	Yes	No
■ Am I asking for help more than I used to?	____	____
■ Am I connecting to a supportive social network?	____	____
■ Am I trying relaxation exercises or mind-body activities to help me revitalize regularly?	____	____
■ Am I clearing clutter at home and at work?	____	____

Pessimistic Thinker

Weight Busters
Realize Pessimism's Perils

On their initial visits, it's quite common for pessimistic thinkers to tell me that they're beyond help and that nobody has ever been able to help them lose weight. If your attitude is similar, let me say that I truly believe that I can help anyone—that is, if you let me. So the question here is not how can I help you but *how can you let me* help you. First, the good news is that instead of being a genetic trait, pessimism is a learned habit that can be broken. So if you think about your pessimistic attitude as being an obstacle that has gotten between you and successful weight loss, I am here to help you break through that barrier. And you can start by opening your eyes, ears, and heart to the following ways that pessimism interferes with your ability to lose weight:

■ It wastes precious time and energy that could be used toward helping yourself.
■ It clouds your mind with so much negativity that weight loss seems to be an impossible task.
■ It impairs your self-confidence.
■ It can become a self-fulfilling prophecy as negative thinking encourages negative outcomes.
■ Just like stress, it negatively affects both your physical and mental health and compromises the immune system, making you more prone to illness.

Think about how your pessimism keeps your mood low. Are you always dissatisfied and arguing with yourself? Redirect those negative energies toward positive outcomes, and it will help you shed the pounds. Once you admit that the pessimistic attitude only worsens your problems, the following steps can lead you to workable solutions.

Turn "I Can't" into "I Can"

If you say "I can't" to every new strategy for losing weight, then you're cinching your fate, because you're not even willing to be a player in the weight loss game. Attempting to turn "I can't" into "I can" declares that you're willing to take a chance and play—even if it is by someone else's rules. But since a can-do attitude is something that doesn't come naturally to you, I'll show you a cognitive restructuring technique, called reframing, that will make it easier.

> ➤ *Nibble on This* ⇐
>
> "Seeing things from a different and more flexible perspective is a great tool to have in your mental bag of tricks."
>
> —DR. JOAN BORYSENKO, *INNER PEACE FOR BUSY PEOPLE*

There are many different ways to look at or think about the same reality. For example, if you quit your job, does that mean you were a failure or that you finally had the strength to find something better? You see, when you choose a view that's less stressful, not only does your outlook improve, but so can your outcome. Reframing encourages you to look at your problems as opportunities, not obstacles. It also supports the underlying notion that you can control the way you respond to things.

Reframing Technique

Pessimistic Thoughts ("I can't")	Reframed Thoughts ("I can")
"This will never work."	"Just as this program has helped many other people, it can help me too."
"I can't keep a food diary."	"People who keep food diaries have been shown to lose more weight than the ones who didn't. Why fight something that's been proved to work?"
"Even if I lose weight, I'll gain it back."	"I'll never know unless I try."

Reframing is a skill that takes some practice. Your first challenge is to listen to your thoughts so you are able to capture them. If writing them down helps you, then do so. And when you hear them (for example, "Even if I lose weight, I'll gain it back"), you can try using the STOP method for taking back control and refocusing: S—slow down, T—take a breath, O—observe objectively without attitude or emotion, P—plan a different response—which may be, "I'll never know unless I try." Think about each time that you devise a more constructive way to look at a situation as being another step taken toward weight loss and improved health. With time, your confidence, outlook, and outcome will improve.

> ⮞ *Nibble on This* ⮜
>
> "When the mind quiets down, the body follows suit."
>
> —DR. HERBERT BENSON WITH MARG STARK, *TIMELESS HEALING*

Accentuate the Positive

Successful weight loss occurs when you're able to sustain a combination of positive eating, exercise, and coping strategies that add up over time. Sustaining these behaviors takes motivation and commitment, which for pessimists can be lacking at times. That's why it's important for you to pay attention to the many different measures of success, weight loss being only one of them. And though you may think that it's the best measure, it often occurs more slowly than the other changes that can occur in your mood, energy level, and stamina. So if you write down the many health benefits you experience, you will be accentuating the positive and motivating yourself to stay with the program.

Pay more attention to any positive strategies that you're able to do—leaving uneaten food on your plate because you know you've had enough, taking a mindful walk after dinner, bringing half of your entrée home from the restaurant. Though you may be more used to feeling drained because of your negative focus and thoughts on all you've done wrong, this positive focus will energize you as it promotes a more balanced and positive perspective. Use a scale of 0 percent to 99 percent to predict how satisfying certain activities will be (for example, taking a yoga or exercise class, trying a new healthy recipe), where 0 percent is completely unsatisfactory and 99 percent is totally satisfying. At the completion of the activity, record how satisfying it turned out to be. If things don't turn out as well as you hoped, this exercise helps you to realize that partial success is okay—and much better for the psyche than focusing on complete failure.

The last aspect of accentuating the positive has to do with using humor or lightening up by renting a funny movie, or thinking about how Robin Williams or Jerry Seinfeld would react if he was in your shoes, or just calling a friend who makes you laugh. Humor can be a great tension releaser for everyone, but especially for pessimists who tend to take themselves too seriously. A keen sense of humor helped Peggy better deal with her weight issues. Once she told me she was ready to offer her body to science, saying she would love to be "put in a coma and then wake up 50 pounds lighter." I said I would keep her in mind if such a research study opportunity ever arose. Another time when her pessimistic thoughts seemed to be getting the best of her, I helped her to isolate her pessimistic side (we called it "pessimistic Peggy") or that alien creature who kept trying to tarnish her successes. With time, Peggy learned to "hear" pessimistic Peggy with a new and different voice, one she could laugh at and discuss as an evil force that could be conquered.

Treat Yourself Better

Pessimistic thinkers can have trouble realizing that they deserve to be treated better. That's because the negativity that causes them to focus on all their failures can also make them overlook all their successes. The first step here is to focus on the good stuff in your life that you've tended to pass over by making a list of your positive qualities that you are most proud of (like Beth's self-affirmations on pages 132–133). Take whatever time you need to complete your list. If this is hard for you to do alone, ask someone you trust for help. I recommend that you read this list over regularly and even carry it with you. Once you start believing in yourself, you'll be in a better place to treat yourself better, from the heart—because you'll know you deserve it.

The concept of self-nurturance may be new to you. What it means is that you care for yourself—in ways that only you appreciate. Make a list of nonfood activities that you would enjoy doing and think about ways you can build these activities into your life. Here are some ideas to get you started.

- Browse in a bookstore.
- Buy yourself some flowers.
- Listen to relaxation tape.
- Listen to music you enjoy.
- Have a spa day at home.
- Buy fancy underwear or sexy lingerie.
- Take a walk in the park.
- Soak in a Jacuzzi.
- Get a free makeover.
- Watch the sunset.
- Get a massage.
- Lie on a hammock and read a good book.

One patient found that a relaxing walk in the park was her ideal way to treat herself, whereas another found that time alone in his favorite easy chair reading a great book worked for him. What matters most is not which activity you choose but that you choose something regularly that you enjoy and that relaxes both your body and your mind.

Success Boosters

Now that you better understand how pessimism impairs your progress, you're putting forth effort to turn "I can't" into "I can." Accentuating the positive and affirming yourself encourage greater self-nurturance. Check your progress with these questions:

	Yes	No
Am I able to admit that pessimism only worsens my problems?	____	____
Am I trying to turn "I can't" into "I can"?	____	____
Is the reframing technique helping me to do so?	____	____
Am I paying attention to other measures of success besides just weight loss?	____	____
Am I focusing on positive strategies that I'm able to carry out?	____	____
Am I using humor?	____	____

■ Do my self-affirmations help me to focus on my
positive qualities?   ____   ____
■ Did I make a list of self-nurturing activities I
would enjoy?   ____   ____

Unrealistic Achiever

Weight Busters
Trim Goals

Whether it's being successful in a business, acquiring an advanced degree, or
raising healthy and productive children, unrealistic achievers are used to
achieving a high degree of success in their lives. But managing their weight has
been different—they just can't get control of it. So when they come to see me
feeling stressed and discouraged, I first help them to tone down their expectations, which in and of itself diminishes their stress.

Wanting them to be successful, I tell them that they need to set a goal
that's practical, realistic, and achievable—I call it the 10 percent goal. For
example, if you currently weigh 175 pounds, then losing 10 percent of 175 or
17.5 pounds would mean that a weight of 157.5 pounds is a realistic goal for
you. Though I know that a goal of losing only 17.5 pounds may be disap-
pointing, I encourage you to think of this as being your first big subgoal. And
once you achieve it, you can set another 10 percent goal. Making these smaller
goals motivates unrealistic achievers to refocus their attentions away from the
emotional struggle of having to lose so much weight and instead toward actually doing something about it.

Focus on the Process

Reaching a goal depends on the process of getting there. Focusing on the
process is nothing new to the business world or, for that matter, to my program. And though I'm not advocating throwing away your weight scale, I
do advocate not using it as your sole focus or motivator for this program.

If you find yourself discouraged and feel that you're not losing enough
weight or not losing it fast enough, turning your focus onto the weight buster
strategies will keep your weight loss efforts moving in the right direction. But
focusing on the process works only if you can step outside your comfort zone

and be willing to take some risks. Depending on your diet personality profile, this may mean ordering new foods at your favorite restaurant, taking your dog for longer walks in the neighborhood, or asking for help. Unrealistic achievers who are used to being successful need to understand that if you do these things, small setbacks are to be expected. So you may not like every new food you taste, or you may not always have time to walk your dog longer, or asking for help may not always work. But that doesn't signal that it's time to stop trying or to give up. As you strive for progress, not perfection, you'll learn that setbacks are not the end of the world or a reason to abandon your program. Instead, they are just signs that you need to be flexible. So if one strategy doesn't work, learn why and then just try another one.

Redirect Energies

Now that you've got your realistic subgoals and you're focusing on the process, weight loss is occurring, but don't be surprised if it's not fast enough for you. It never is for unrealistic achievers. To counteract your tendency to feel stressed or discouraged, keep your energy positive by refocusing it on your other life passions. Complete a life passions inventory (see page 143) and think about things in your life that you have always wanted to do but never had the time. Make the time for something that's important to you. This exercise helps to remind you that your life is more than what you weigh. And being able to focus on relationship, work, spiritual, or self-care passions helps to put weight loss in a more realistic perspective. One patient who had already lost 15 pounds decided to take kayaking lessons as a way of recapturing his feelings of youth and adventure. For him, following a life passion had a secondary benefit of burning more calories and advancing his weight loss even farther. Another patient took a gourmet cooking class that she later could apply to preparing healthier meals for her and her family. What was refreshing was that through thinking about their life passions, both patients furthered their weight loss but without having to work so hard.

> ⮞ *Nibble on This* ⮜
> Take a break from trying so hard. It may be just what you need.

Accept Limitations

You're following the outlined strategies and you've been steadily losing weight. But some unrealistic achievers would still like to mold their bodies into something that they're not, which means they're still not satisfied. That's when I discuss their genetic or biological limitations that form their non-negotiables of weight loss. Though 60–65 percent of your weight is unrelated to genetics, that means that 35–40 percent of your weight is genetically determined. For example, if many members of your extended family have a weight problem, then maybe some of your problems are also genetic. The same holds true for the distribution of your weight, particularly in your hips, thighs, and buttocks. And as hormones shift for postmenopausal women, fat deposits also shift from the hips, thighs, and buttocks to the abdomen. Though lifestyle changes can counteract midlife weight gain by building muscle mass to speed metabolism, biology prevents you from counteracting all of your genetic factors.

The bottom line is that you can still be successful in achieving your healthier lifestyle behaviors yet be unable to perfectly mold or carve your body into your beauty ideal. And when it comes down to predicting your health 10 years from now, the most important predictor is NOT whether you manage to lose 10 more pounds. Rather, it's how fit you are, how active you are every day, how healthy your diet is, and how you cope with the stresses of daily living. Learning to accept these limitations allows the unrealistic achiever to accept successes and progress, take pride in a healthier lifestyle—and then move on.

> ⇒ *Nibble on This* ⇐
>
> "Healthy bodies come in all shapes and sizes."
>
> —DR. STEVEN BLAIR, EPIDEMIOLOGIST, COOPER INSTITUTE FOR AEROBICS RESEARCH, DALLAS

Success Boosters

Now that you're trimming your weight loss goals to make them more realistic, you're better able to focus on the process of weight loss. And knowing that setbacks are a part of the process, being flexible helps you to take some risks and learn new things. The process of accepting your biological limitations helps you focus on staying active, eating healthier, and coping better with stress, which are your best health predictors. Check your progress with these questions:

	Yes	No
■ Are more realistic subgoals helping me to focus my program?	___	___
■ Is focusing on the process helping me to better achieve my goals?	___	___
■ Is my flexibility helping me to better deal with minor setbacks?	___	___
■ Is redirecting my energies helping me to broaden my focus in life?	___	___
■ Am I working toward accepting my limitations?	___	___

■ ■ ■ ■ ■

Chapter 6

Staying on Track

The strategies throughout this book have shown that you can take back control of your weight by comfortably and confidently taking charge of your eating, exercise, and coping habits. But getting there is only half the battle; keeping your authentic shape is the real goal. If you're a chronic dieter, this goal has eluded you. But not anymore. The good news is that unlike most one-dimensional, restrictive diets you've been on in the past, this book's weight maintenance strategies are the same as the ones you've already been using throughout the book—with one important distinction. Successful weight maintenance requires a three-step process: (1) periodic self-monitoring, (2) troubleshooting, and (3) taking corrective action. This is a fluid process whereby you learn to adapt weight loss strategies to your changing life challenges and diet personality patterns. Though over time your patterns can shift, common threads or core behaviors (that are consistent with the guidelines of the American Heart Association, the USDA, the American College of Sports Medicine, and the principles of cognitive behavioral therapy) anchor this program and run throughout all of the patterns. Highlighting these behaviors will remind you of the fundamental strategies learned throughout the book—that are sure to keep you focused on the healthy weight loss track.

Periodic Self-Monitoring

Self-monitoring is the key to long-term weight control. When patients come back to my program after a prolonged absence, they invariably tell me that the very first thing that derailed their success was that they stopped using a self-monitoring tool. Whether it was weighing themselves, recording their diet, or wearing a pedometer, the less they monitored, the more weight they gained and the worse they felt. By periodically monitoring or inventorying your patterns, you can stay on track and prevent lapses from turning into collapses.

> *Nibble on This* <

The National Weight Control Registry shows that of a group of individuals who have been extremely successful weight loss maintainers, more than 44 percent weigh themselves at least once a day and 31 percent weigh themselves at least once a week.

In addition to weighing yourself regularly (I recommend weekly), use the progress tracking form below monthly. Amy found that a monthly monitoring tool was just enough to remind her to stay on track and to warn her of an impending lapse in behaviors. And pairing this activity with paying her monthly bills made it easy for her to remember. It was just about six months into the program when Amy had reached her weight goal (having lost 35 pounds). Amy's sample progress tracking form on pages 165–166 shows how she progressed from there.

Progress Tracking Form

Date					
Eating Patterns					
Unguided Grazer					
Nighttime Nibbler					
Convenient Consumer					
Fruitless Feaster					
Mindless Muncher					
Hearty Portioner					
Deprived Sneaker					
Exercise Patterns					
Hate-to-Move Struggler					
Self-Conscious Hider					
Inexperienced Novice					
All-or-Nothing Doer					
Set-Routine Repeater					
Aches-and-Pains Sufferer					
No-Time-to-Exercise Protester					
Coping Patterns					
Emotional Stuffer					
Low-Self-Esteem Sufferer					

Progress Tracking Form (cont.)

Date								
Coping Patterns								
Persistent Procrastinator								
Can't-Say-No Pleaser								
Fast Pacer								
Pessimistic Thinker								
Unrealistic Achiever								
Overall Progress Self-Evaluation								
Weight								

Amy's Progress Tracking Form

Date	Sept. 1	Oct. 1	Nov. 1	Nov. 8	Nov. 15	Nov. 22
Eating Patterns						
Unguided Grazer	90%	70%	60%			
Nighttime Nibbler						
Convenient Consumer						
Fruitless Feaster						
Mindless Muncher						
Hearty Portioner						
Deprived Sneaker	80%	60%	60%			
Exercise Patterns						
Hate-to-Move Struggler						
Self-Conscious Hider						
Inexperienced Novice						
All-or-Nothing Doer						
Set-Routine Repeater						
Aches-and-Pains Sufferer						
No-Time-to-Exercise Protester	70%	60%	20%			
Coping Patterns						
Emotional Stuffer	60%	50%	10%			
Low-Self-Esteem Sufferer						

Amy's Progress Tracking Form (cont.)

Date	Sept. 1	Oct. 1	Nov. 1	Nov. 8	Nov. 15	Nov. 22
Coping Patterns						
Persistent Procrastinator						
Can't-Say-No Pleaser						
Fast Pacer						
Pessimistic Thinker						
Unrealistic Achiever						
Overall Progress Self-Evaluation	70%	60%	25%			
Weight	150 lbs.	152 lbs.	155 lbs.			

The percents indicate how well Amy shaped her symptom patterns. Compared with her initial success in controlling her patterns, Amy's patterns began slipping in October, and they worsened by November. This "pattern recidivism" was associated with a 5-pound weight gain over the 2 months. This "drifting away from the program" was an all-too-familiar theme for Amy that followed all previous weight control attempts. But this time would be different. Instead of giving up, the slip in behaviors prompted Amy to reinstitute weekly monitoring. She knew the warning signs that signaled it was time to start troubleshooting:

- an abrupt decline in self-rating scores
- a slow, steady decline in self-rating scores
- a 5-pound weight gain

Troubleshooting

The process of troubleshooting involves taking a close look at a situation and trying to understand the reason for the change in behavior. In Amy's case, the loss of control of her patterns was triggered by moving to the suburbs and spending more time commuting to and from work. Though her eating patterns remained under control, her exercise and coping routines were now disrupted—and her progress tracking form showed it. Troubleshooting for Amy meant reanalyzing her patterns in light of the changes in her home and work environments. Old habits were reemerging. The no-time-to-exercise protester pattern was more prevalent than ever since she now spent 40 extra minutes driving to and from work. And she also found herself turning to food for comfort during her stressful and long commute. This was consistent with her pattern of being an emotional stuffer. By analyzing the reasons for her weight gain, for the first time Amy was *not blaming herself* for her failure. The causes were apparent and understandable. She was ready to take corrective action—the third step for long-term weight control.

If control of your strategies begins to lapse, the reasons will become evident by conducting a careful analysis of your lifestyle. Chances are that a new or recurring pressure from scaling up syndrome is the cause. Some of the reasons will be short-lived and predictable, such as tax season for an accountant or having houseguests for the holidays. The goal here is to be aware of and pay attention to the influences these changes have on your patterns, and to resume the scaling down strategies as soon as you possibly can. However, if the lifestyle change is either long-term or permanent, such as a change in job, residence, or relationship, then a more formal review of your personality patterns is in order. I discuss developing new patterns later in this chapter.

Taking Corrective Action

Identifying the problems leads directly to taking action. Amy reviewed the strategies and applied new solutions to her new problems.

- Regarding her no-time-to-exercise protester pattern, once Amy began wearing her pedometer daily, she felt much more in control of her activity level. Within a few weeks, she was able to build 10,000 steps back into her day. Amy also came to the realization that with this new commuting schedule, weekday trips to the health club were unrealistic. So she purchased a home treadmill, which she now uses 4 mornings a week before going to work. Sure, she has to get up earlier, but being active makes her feel so much better that she says it's well worth the effort.
- Regarding her emotional stuffer pattern, Amy completed a new ABC food/mood behavior chain diary and saw that feelings of loneliness were triggering this new onset of emotional eating. Amy acknowledged that she missed her friends and active social life in the city. So she developed an emotional eating action plan that consisted of calling old friends and scheduling regular outings with them, meeting new friends at work, and making an effort to meet her new neighbors. Instead of reaching out for food, Amy began reaching out socially. She also got some books on tape from the library to make her long commute less stressful and more enjoyable.
- Within 4 weeks, Amy had lost 3 of the 5 pounds she had previously gained and was back on track.

To recommit yourself to the program and get control of drifting patterns, it is often useful to keep a diary again for a few days and to institute other self-monitoring tools such as wearing a pedometer, paying more attention to food labels, weighing yourself regularly, or even using the progress tracking form weekly. You also might talk to someone you trust about the difficulties you are having and what he or she can do to help. The more support you have around you, the more successful you will be. And don't be discouraged that you are having a lapse in your program. That is to be expected due to changes in lifestyle, personal priorities, and unpredictable situations.

Recognizing New Patterns

If you've taken the corrective actions that have gotten your present patterns under control, but you're still gaining weight, you may have developed a new pattern. This means that a more formal review of your personality patterns is in order. Either take the diet personality quiz again or read over the pattern descriptions in Chapter 2. The key to success here is recognizing a developing pattern early enough so you can implement its strategies and take back control. I use the following three patient scenarios for illustration:

- At 48 years old, Iris was thrilled about her progress, having lost 20 pounds in 4 months, maintaining the loss for 6 months, and feeling that all of her patterns were under control. Then she broke her leg in a skiing accident and everything changed. Instead of attending aerobics classes, Iris found herself going to physical therapy and struggling to walk. Though frustrated at first because her complete fitness routine had been disrupted, she decided to step back, reevaluate her situation, and take charge of the new pattern she realized she developed: the aches-and-pains sufferer. Iris tackled the new strategies head-on as rehabilitating her leg back to full function became her new fitness goal, outlined by her physician. While waiting for her injured leg to heal, Iris's therapist gave her a resistance-training program so she could continue to build the strength of her upper body and maintain the strength of her good leg. Because Iris identified this new pattern early on, her weight gain during this setback was a mere 3 pounds that she eventually was able to lose once her cast was removed and she resumed full activities.
- Ava's experience was quite different, as she had been able to enjoy only 1 week of being at her weight loss goal of 140 pounds, when her father had become quite ill. It seemed that almost overnight, the time that Ava had been spending on her own self-care was now filled with chaffeuring,

going to and from doctor appointments, and just being with her parents. Though Ava's siblings all lived nearby, Ava found herself solely caring for her parents, never asking anyone else for help, and feeling resentful about it. Ava came in to see me, desperate for help as she knew she was relapsing but didn't know how to get back on track. I helped Ava to realize that she had developed the can't-say-no-pleaser coping pattern and she needed to take back control—which she did. She took this time to think about the yeses in her life (that had changed) and to ask her siblings for help so she could make them happen. Ava wanted to spend a lot of time with her parents, but she also needed a "mental health" break now and then. These breaks allowed her to get back to exercise, which was a great tension reliever, and to connect spiritually by spending time with her mom at their church. By asking for help, Ava was coping better, and though her weight gain still fluctuated between 2 and 5 pounds, she was satisfied, given the stress she was under.

■ For Doug, a 56-year-old marketing executive who had lost 12 pounds over 3 months by taking total control of his convenient consumer eating pattern, weight maintenance was going quite well. But things abruptly changed when Doug's company merged with another one and he was promoted to vice president. Suddenly Doug was juggling so many roles that by the end of the day, he had nothing left for himself. Though Doug was happy about this promotion, he felt distracted and stressed most of the time. These feelings prompted Doug to talk to his wife and get help. Together they realized that Doug had become a fast pacer and needed to take action. Recognizing the imbalances in his life was the first step, and following this pattern's mindfulness and relaxation strategies was the second. Doug also pared down his responsibilities by hiring a much-needed personal assistant. It took 6 to 8 weeks before Doug could honestly say that he was feeling like his old self. And his weight showed it as he was able to lose the few pounds he had gained back.

These scenarios help support my beliefs about how to handle your weight maintenance goals at these difficult times of life:

■ Whenever you're in the midst of a life crisis, you need to give yourself a break.

- Until the crisis passes, set a new goal either to maintain your weight or keep weight gain under 5 pounds.
- At the very least, make time to get support, either from a friend, family member, health professional, member of the clergy, support group, book, or even from a chat room on the Internet.
- Hold on to the core behaviors below that are fundamental to your healthier lifestyle.

Keeping Core Behaviors

A review of the following eating, exercise, and coping core behaviors that form the basis for my patterns approach will help you to stay on track.

Select Super Foods

"Super Foods" are a dieter's dream, a class of plant foods that our research dietitian identified to provide maximum nutritional value for relatively minimal calories. A cornucopia of super foods is available throughout our dietary landscape, some being staples of our diet while others being less common. Since Americans typically select higher-fat and -calorie foods with less nutritional value, they have limited experiences cooking with and enjoying super foods.

Super foods are exclusively plant-based foods—fruits, vegetables, grains, nuts, seeds, dried beans, lentils, or soy products—that are generally low to moderate in fat and calories but are naturally rich in vitamins, minerals, fiber, and disease-fighting phytochemicals (see Chapter 7 for more information). For example, collard greens are a super food because a half-cup portion of cooked greens contains only 25 calories and a significant amount of folate, calcium, and fiber, and is a "super" dietary source of vitamins A and C. For a weight-reducing diet, collard greens are a nutritional powerhouse. The super recipes in Chapter 7, which all contain at least one super food ingredient, show you how to incorporate more super foods (like collard greens) into your diet.

> *Dieting Myth: Carbohydrates make you fat.*
> Carbophobia or fear of carbohydrates causes some people to avoid fresh fruits and vegetables and to skip whole-grain breads and pastas. In the right portions (and without high-fat toppings or sauces), these complex, high-fiber carbohydrates are an important and satisfying component of healthy weight loss.

Studies have shown that obesity is relatively rare in populations that consume a high-fiber diet rich in super foods. The reason is that fiber makes it easier to reduce dietary calories, and that's the key to losing weight. Although it's not a magic bullet, fiber is about as close as you will get. Its bulking properties make you feel fuller and more satisfied. Additional benefits include improved blood sugar control (for diabetics), lowered blood cholesterol, reduced risk of heart disease and some forms of cancer, and less constipation. I recommend getting fiber from natural foods instead of from dietary supplements since it's the best way to build a healthy diet. Fiber comes only from plant sources—whole-grain products, fruits, and vegetables. Try to consume 25–38 grams per day (that is nearly double the amount that the average American currently consumes). To reach this target, I recommend substituting whole-grain products for refined ones and choosing more fruits and vegetables with each meal and snack.

Another benefit to eating super foods is that they're low to moderate in energy density, which is a nutrition bonus for those needing to eat fewer calories to promote weight loss. Energy density is not a familiar term to the average dieter—but it needs to be. It turns out that your sense of fullness and contentment is actually gauged after you eat some amount or volume of food rather than after consuming a defined number of calories. In other words, if you are served a large bowl of spaghetti on two consecutive nights, one night with tomato sauce and vegetables (higher-fiber, lower-calorie super foods) and the other with a cream sauce (higher calorie), you are likely to eat about the same amount each night even though one dish had many more calories. There is something about the sight and physical sensation of the volume of food consumed that is important to feeling full. So if you choose your foods wisely, you can fill up and feel satisfied with fewer calories.

By definition, foods lower in energy density have fewer calories per given weight than do foods higher in energy density. The combination of elements in a food—fat, carbohydrate, protein, fiber, and water—determines energy density. As a general rule, the higher the water content, the lower the energy density. That's why most fruits, vegetables, and broth-based soups are low calorie and very filling. The same holds true for many cooked grains, breakfast cereals with low-fat milk, low-fat meats, beans, and salads. At the other end of the spectrum are foods high in energy density—crackers, chips, cookies, doughnuts, and butter. These foods are very high in calories with little in the way of fullness in return. The following table gives examples of less-calorie-dense meals you can try.

Less-Calorie-Dense Meals

Old Meals	New Meals (Less Calorie-Dense)
Old Breakfasts	New Breakfasts
Low-fiber cereal, whole milk	High-fiber cereal or hot oatmeal with brown sugar, skim milk, red grapefruit
Fried eggs and bacon	Scrambled egg whites, whole wheat toast, extralean ham, sliced strawberries
Cheese omelet and sausage	Egg white omelet with mushrooms, onions, and light mozzarella or soy cheese, soy "sausage" link
Jelly doughnut, coffee	High-fiber bagel, light cream cheese or Laughing Cow cheese, honeydew melon, coffee
Fast-food French toast sticks, orange juice	Whole-grain toaster waffles, sliced orange, low-fat milk
Old Lunches	New Lunches
Salami sandwich and potato chips	Lean turkey sandwich on whole-grain bread, lettuce and tomato, mustard; fresh fruit salad
Chili dog and french fries	Vegetarian chili and side green lettuce salad
Cream of chicken soup and crackers	Bean or vegetable soup and whole-grain crackers
Cheeseburger and fried onion rings	Veggie burger on whole-grain bun with tomato, lettuce, pickle, and barbecue sauce; coleslaw
Yogurt and pretzels	Reduced-fat cottage cheese mixed with yogurt and sliced peaches; high-fiber crispbread
Old Dinners	New Dinners
Fried fish and french fried onion rings	Grilled fish, vegetable stir-fry over brown rice, whole-grain bread
Chicken wings and potato chips	Skinless dark chicken, roasted potatoes, and vegetables; minestrone soup

Barbecued ribs, french fries, and corn	Barbecued chicken, baked sweet potato wedges, noncreamy coleslaw
Fettucini Alfredo and garlic bread	Whole wheat spiral pasta with olive oil, garlic, broccoli, and parmesan cheese or topped with marinara sauce; large salad with low-fat dressing
Breaded pork chop, creamed spinach	Vegetable and pork stir-fry over rice; spinach salad

Increase Omega 3s and Monounsaturated Heart-Healthy Fats

Omega-3 fats are found in fatty fish and some nuts and seeds, such as walnuts and flaxseed. These oils have been shown to reduce heart disease and improve immune function. The other oil that is reasonable to add to your diet (in moderation) is monounsaturated fat, like olive oil and canola oil. Keep in mind, though, that all fats contain 9 calories per gram. That's why I recommend using monounsaturated fat as a condiment for flavor and taste. So instead of snacking on walnuts, I suggest you enjoy them sprinkled on salads or stir-fry dishes.

Dieting Myth: Avoid all fat.

Fatphobia, or the fear of fat, causes some of you to overeat fat-free foods (that are almost equal in calories to their full-fat counterparts, high in sugar, and low in satiety) and to eat few heart-healthy fats—both poor recipes for a satisfying weight loss program. Heart-healthy polyunsaturated and monoun-saturated fats found in avocados, walnuts, salmon, and olive oil enhance the flavor, aroma, moisture, and taste of many foods.

Eat Lean Protein

Including protein in your diet is essential for good health, particularly while you are actively losing weight. But your protein sources should not all be animal-based—from meat, fish, poultry, and dairy products. These foods are often laden with fat and calories and, despite containing a significant amount of nutrients, they do not contain any fiber or phytochemicals. They're not considered super foods.

If you are like most Americans, your protein consumption probably exceeds the recommended dietary allowance (RDA) of 0.4 gram per pound of body weight. That equates to about 65 grams for a 160-pound individual and 80 grams for a 200-pound person. Overall, protein should make up about 10 to 35 percent of total calories, according to the latest guidelines from the Institute of Medicine. My recommendation here is threefold. First, if you eat animal protein, choose lean trimmed meats, skimmed dairy products, skinless poultry, fish, and egg whites. The only recommended exception to this rule is fish, which can be fatty since it contains omega 3s (as previously discussed). Second, be sure to include ample amounts of vegetable proteins in your diet. Everyday super food sources include soy (tofu, soy milk, edamame, meat substitutes, Luna bars), lentils, beans, nuts, grains, and other vegetables. Soy is particularly healthy to add to your diet since it contains cancer- and heart disease–fighting phytochemicals. And third, include a protein source with each of your meals. Protein is important for energy and reduces your hunger following meals.

Dieting Myth: You need meat protein in a diet to be healthy.
Sure, we all need some protein in our diet, especially when cutting overall calories and losing weight. The confusion comes when people think that meat is the preferred or only source. Less and lean should be your motto when it comes to eating meat. Fish and vegetable protein sources (beans, lentils, nuts, and soy) are healthy options that add *fewer calories but more variety and good taste* to a weight loss program. So there are many reasons to say "Where's the beef?" less often.

Drink More Water

Since water is the very substance we are made of (73 percent of our lean tissue is water), it needs to be frequently replenished. The more hydrated you keep yourself, the more energetic you will feel. I tout water for two additional reasons. If you have fallen into the habit of drinking juices and regular colas as your preferred beverages, you're drinking hundreds of calories each day, and that alone can make the difference between losing and not losing weight. Switching to water immediately eliminates these unneeded, extra calories. The second reason is that dehydration is often misinterpreted as hunger. So instead of turning to water and quenching your thirst, you may be eating food instead. If you keep yourself hydrated, it is likely to help control your total calorie intake. How much water do you need? Although water requirements vary depending on how much you weigh and how active you are, the general rule of thumb is 64 ounces (8 glasses) daily.

Decrease Saturated and Trans Fats

This is the first recommendation where I am advising you to *reduce* something rather than add. The reason is that saturated and trans fats are "killer fats" and have no role in a healthy diet. Saturated fats are found in whole dairy and fatty meat products and in many prepared bakery foods. Trans fats are primarily made by artificially hardening vegetable oils into margarines. They are also found in many savory snack foods. By ridding your diet of these fats, you will not only be eating more "heart healthy" but also cutting calories from your diet. To put this recommendation into action, choose only skimmed dairy products and lean meats, and check all food labels for saturated and trans fats (hydrogenated oils on the food label signify that trans fats are in the product).

Turn up Your Calorie Meter

Your body is continuously burning calories and never stops, each and every 1,440 minutes in a day. The amount of calories burned is a function of your age (the younger you are, the more calories you burn), your weight (the heavier you are, the more calories you burn), and most important, how active you are—this last determinant being entirely under your control (versus weight, which is about 60 percent under your control and the remainder thought to be genetics).

Increasing the amount of calories burned through ADLs (activities of daily living, the sum of all the body movements you make over the course of the day) and aerobics (scheduled exercise) is the basis of my exercise strategies. When it comes to long-term weight loss, physical activity is the most significant predictor of success.

> ⇌ *Nibble on This* ⇋
>
> If you are overweight, you should engage in a minimum of 150 minutes of moderate-intensity activity (continuous housecleaning, aerobic or resistance exercise) per week, but for long-term weight loss, you need to progress to more than 200 minutes.

Continuously advancing your physical activity routine is also essential because your body adapts to familiar and repeated movements. Regardless of what you are doing, regularly change the pace, duration, intensity, or frequency. This will challenge your muscles and enhance cardiorespiratory fitness.

> *Dieting Myth: If I exercise, I can eat whatever I want and lose weight.*
> Some of my patients have been exercising 3–4 times a week for months but are exasperated because they've been losing minimal or no weight at all. In fact, many are convinced that their bodies just do not work. The truth is that food calories have a much greater impact on your body weight equation (especially at the beginning of a weight loss program) than exercise does. Here's why. If you replace your usual nighttime snack of a 340-calorie Dove Bar with a 45-calorie fruit juice bar, you just saved yourself 295 calories. In contrast, if you walk on a treadmill for 30 minutes, you burn about 115 calories (depending on your weight and exercise intensity) above your resting calories. So calorie for calorie, you get more "bang for your buck" by cutting back on food calories. This shouldn't be confused with the fact that exercising long term is one of the best predictors of a dieter's ability to maintain weight loss. So though exercise is vitally important to a healthy weight loss program, food strategies must be added for the maximum weight loss benefit.

Rev Up Your Metabolism

Trying to lose and maintain weight without strength training is like trying to play catch with one hand tied behind your back—it can be done, but it is a lot easier if you use both hands. The reason strength training is so important to dieters is that it increases basal metabolic rate, or BMR. Since BMR is primarily determined by how muscular you are, building muscle allows you to burn more calories even at rest! Resistance training has other health benefits, including improved strength, endurance, muscle tone, and bone density. Strive for 2 to 3 days per week on nonconsecutive days to allow your muscles to rest. If you think you have a sluggish metabolism, chances are you have not included resistance training into your routine.

Enjoy the Spillover Benefits of Exercise

So much about losing weight comes down to how you feel about yourself, how your body feels, and the confidence in your ability to succeed. A wonderful spillover benefit of exercise is the empowerment that you feel from being a physically active person. Studies have shown that exercise improves mood, reduces depression, and relieves stress. And once you feel your mood lift with exercise, you are more motivated to remain physically active.

Take Time to Destress

It's no secret that stress can be a powerful trigger to overeating. Some researchers even cite stress hormones as causing abdominal fat deposition in women. Stress has also been proved to make people more susceptible to illness and decrease their ability to recover from illness. Yet most diet books offer food-only approaches without addressing this important dimension of weight control. Instead, I feel it's essential for you to confront your false weight/stress connection head-on if you want to lose weight—and keep it off.

Change Your Mind Along with Your Body

Losing weight is about so much more than just carbs, protein, and aerobics—it is also about self-acceptance, self-care, and self-esteem. Your attitudes, emotions, and relationships have a strong impact on your physical health. Researchers have even shown that an optimistic attitude, a strong social network, and spirituality all influence one's health and well-being. Your attitudes also impact your day-to-day decision making, problem solving, and chosen health behaviors—all factors critical to healthy weight loss.

Strengthen Your Mind-Body Connection

Researchers have proved that through the relaxation response, you can learn to cope better with stress and even improve your physical health. Understanding how your mind can relax your body and how your body can relax your mind can have powerful effects on your mood—and your weight. Though many dieters desperately want something external (a pill or "miracle" diet) to jump-start their weight loss, it's actually your internal mind-body strategies that can be a powerful catalyst to feeling better about yourself and taking control of your weight.

Counting Family and Friends

Staying on track is easier when you have a supportive social network. At times it will be useful (or even necessary) to understand the patterns of your family, friends, and coworkers so that you can elicit support and avoid conflict. For example, if your spouse and children are also overweight and you want to make healthier lifestyles a "family affair," it's important to know their patterns so that you can directly address their unique issues. Having fresh fruit around the house, serving vegetables with dinner, and making some meatless meals will support the fruitless feasters in the family. If you and your "lunch bunch" coworkers are mindless munchers, then keeping candy off all of your desks is a mutually winning ticket. And buddying up with fellow hate-to-move strugglers in the neighborhood can get you and your neighbors on the right fitness track. You see, one interesting thing about scaling up syndrome is that it can have an effect on everyone around you. And others are bound to join in and scale down—once you show them the way.

■　　■　　■　　■　　■

Chapter 7

Scaling Down with Super Food Recipes

T hough patients commonly worry that healthy cooking will be a labor-intensive chore, just a few visits with one of my registered dietitians can quickly prove them wrong. Your grandmother may have spent endless hours in the kitchen, but you are not your grandmother. Instead, you're probably curious to learn about any flavor-boosting and time-saving tips on the healthy cooking front. Here are the top ten tactics my dietitians and patients have found helpful. I hope you will too.

Healthy Cooking and Grocery Shopping Tips

Stock Your Kitchen with Post-Its

Most people don't need an intricate organizational system to ensure that their kitchen stays stocked with healthy foods for the coming week—all they need are Post-its. As you finish your last carton of yogurt, eat your last orange, sprinkle the last dash of a favorite seasoning, or finish the box of a favorite healthy snack food, jot the item on a large Post-it, stick it to a counter or the side of the refrigerator, and keep it as your running list. Encourage family members to add to it. Each week, quickly check the levels of your healthy staples (see three-week starter plan's sample shopping list in Appendix B), list the ingredients needed for one or two new recipes, grab your Post-it, and you're good to go grocery shopping.

> ➢ *Nibble on This* ☙
>
> "Your diet is only as healthy as your last trip to the grocery store."
>
> —DAWN JACKSON, REGISTERED DIETITIAN, NORTHWESTERN MEMORIAL HOSPITAL WELLNESS INSTITUTE

Be a Savvy Shopper

A savvy shopper quickly deciphers food labels as well as navigates the grocery store aisles. Below, I highlight the most important label features when it comes to healthy weight loss. Getting comfortable with label reading can begin in your own kitchen and then continue on your shopping trips. Once you understand label-reading basics, you'll be surprised at how quickly you can sharpen this skill. The three-step process of label reading can become a quick, one-step process of comparing calories and serving sizes. Doing a "head to head" comparison between two products can help you make the decision between what goes in your cart—and stomach—and what stays on the grocery shelf.

Label 1

Label 2

Label 1

Nutrition Facts

Serving Size 2 crackers (14g)
Servings Per Carton about 17

Amount Per Serving

Calories 60   Calories from Fat 10

% Daily Value*

Total Fat 1.5g	**2%**
Saturated Fat 0g	**0%**
Polyunsaturated Fat 1g	
Monounsaturated Fat 0g	
Cholesterol 0mg	**0%**
Sodium 90mg	**4%**
Total Carbohydrate 10g	**3%**
Dietary Fiber 3g	**13%**
Sugars 0g	
Other Carbohydrate 7g	
Protein 1g	

Vitamin A 0%	•	Vitamin C 0%
Calcium 0%	•	Iron 2%

*Percent Daily Values are based on a 2,000 calorie diet. Your daily values may be higher or lower depending on your calorie needs:

		Calories:	2,000	2,500
Total Fat	Less than		65g	80g
Saturated Fat	Less than		20g	25g
Cholesterol	Less than		300mg	300mg
Sodium	Less than		2,400mg	2,400mg
Total Carbohydrate			300g	375g
Dietary Fiber			25g	30g

Calories per gram:
Fat 9 • Carbohydrate 4 • Protein 4

INGREDIENTS: WHOLE RYE, CORN BRAN, PARTIALLY HYDRO-GENATED SOYBEAN OIL*, SALT, CARAWAY AND BHT (A PRE-SERVATIVE).

*Adds a trivial amount of saturated fat.

Label 2

Nutrition Facts

Serving Size 2 crackers (16g)
Servings Per Container about 21

Amount Per Serving

Calories 70   Calories from Fat 30

% Daily Value*

Total Fat 3.5g	**5%**
Saturated Fat 1g	**5%**
Cholesterol 0mg	**0%**
Sodium 110mg	**5%**
Total Carbohydrate 9g	**3%**
Dietary Fiber 0g	**0%**
Sugars 1g	
Protein 1g	

Vitamin A 0%	•	Vitamin C 0%
Calcium 0%	•	Iron 2%

*Percent Daily Values are based on a 2,000 calorie diet. Your daily values may be higher or lower depending on your calorie needs:

		Calories:	2,000	2,500
Total Fat	Less than		65g	80g
Sat Fat	Less than		20g	25g
Cholesterol	Less than		300mg	300mg
Sodium	Less than		2,400mg	2,400mg
Total Carbohydrate			300g	375g
Dietary Fiber			25g	30g

INGREDIENTS: ENRICHED FLOUR [WHEAT FLOUR, NIACIN, REDUCED IRON, THIAMINE MONONITRATE (VITAMIN B1), RIBOFLAVIN (VITAMIN B2), FOLIC ACID], VEGETABLE SHORTENING (PARTIALLY HYDROGENATED SOYBEAN AND/OR COTTONSEED OIL), SUGAR, BUTTER (CREAM, SALT, ARTIFICIAL COLOR), CONTAINS TWO PERCENT OR LESS OF MALTED BARLEY FLOUR, LEAVENING (SODIUM BICARBONATE, SODIUM ACID PYROPHOSPHATE, MONOCALCIUM PHOSPHATE, YEAST), CORN SYRUP, SALT, HIGH FRUCTOSE CORN SYRUP, SOY LECITHIN.

Three-Step Method for Deciphering a Food Label

Label 1 Features	Quick Facts	Think Like a Nutritionist
Serving size: 2 crackers Calories: 60	1. *Look at the serving size and the calories.* The serving size is at the top of the label. Using common measurements such as pieces, tablespoons, or cups, it is based on the amount of food that people typically eat. All listed nutrients pertain to this serving size.	*Will you eat only one serving?* If you eat double the listed serving size, then you need to double the calories (120), saturated fat, etc. *Look at the calories per serving: is it less than 200 for a snack or 400–600 for a meal?* Decreasing your total calorie intake by about 500 or more per day puts you on the weight loss track.
Dietary fiber: 3g (grams), 13% daily value	2. *Look at the fiber.* Good fiber source products contain 2.5–5 grams of fiber, and high-fiber products contain more than 5 grams. Sometimes a label also tells specifically how much soluble and insoluble fiber are in a product. Both types of fiber are important. Soluble fiber acts more like a *sponge* in the body, helping to lower cholesterol. Insoluble fiber works more like a *broom* in the body, cleaning out the intestinal tract.	*Does the product contain 2.5–5 or more grams of fiber per serving?* A quick guide to the % daily values (which are based on a 2,000-calorie diet): 5% or less means that one serving of this food product is low in that nutrient, and 20% or more means it's high in that nutrient. Because your calorie intake may be more or less than 2,000 calories, use these daily values as references only.
Saturated fat: 0g (grams), 0% daily value Ingredients: partially hydrogenated soybean oil	3. *Look at the unhealthy fats: saturated and trans fats.* Saturated fat is an unhealthy fat that you want to limit in your diet to 10% of your total calories. Someone on a 1,600-calorie diet should eat no more than 16 grams of saturated fat a day. Another unhealthy fat—trans fats—is listed in the ingredients section as "partially hydrogenated oil." Unfortunately it's hard to find a processed snack food without this, though there are some.	*Is the product low in saturated fats (less than or equal to 5% daily value)?* *Is "hydrogenated" or "partially hydrogenated" not present or low on the ingredients list?* Ingredients are listed from the greatest amounts down to the smallest amounts.

Other label facts that may interest you for general health reasons or if you have high cholesterol, high blood pressure, or diabetes:

- Total fat should be less than 35 percent of your *total daily* calories. This takes into account that some foods you eat, like nuts, may be higher in fats, and some foods may be lower. Someone on a 1,600-calorie diet would eat around 50–55 grams of fat per day.

- Cholesterol is found only in animal products. A heart-healthy diet has 300 milligrams of cholesterol or less *per day*. If you have high cholesterol, it's most important to limit saturated fat in your diet. *Reality check: One large whole egg contains 213–220 milligrams of cholesterol, or 71 percent of the daily recommended amount!*

- Protein is recommended to be about 10–35 percent of your daily calories. A person on a 1,600 calorie diet would be eating about 60–80 grams of protein each day. Note: 3 ounces of a chicken breast (the size of a deck of cards) has about 25–30 grams of protein.

- Sodium intake is recommended to be below 2,400 milligrams per day. Only a small amount of sodium naturally occurs in foods. Most sodium is added during processing. So highly processed, prepackaged foods in boxes, in cans, and frozen can have high sodium contents. When reading labels, try to buy products with 480 milligrams sodium or less per serving. *Reality check: 1 teaspoon of salt has 2,300 milligrams of sodium!*

- Sugars on a label are a combination of naturally occurring sugars and added sugars. You need to look at the ingredient list to know if sugars have been added to a product. A food is likely to be high in sugars if a sugar synonym (like high-fructose corn syrup, malt syrup, dextrose, sucrose, or honey) appears first or second on the ingredients list or if several of them are listed. Regular soft drinks, fruit drinks, fat-free foods, candies, cakes, cookies, pies, and many breakfast cereals are high in added sugars. Five or fewer grams of sugar is the equivalent of about 1 teaspoon. *Reality check: 1 can of Pepsi contains 41 grams of sugar, or the equivalent of 8 teaspoons!*

> ➣ *Nibble on This* ➢
>
> "Over the last ten years, the amount of refined, simple sugars used by the food industry has more than doubled. Basically, they've replaced sugar for fat."
>
> —Dr. Linda Van Horn, Professor of Preventive Medicine, Northwestern University

Now that you know how to read between the lines of food labels, there are just a couple more things you need to become a truly savvy shopper. First and foremost, make a commitment to your health to avoid grocery shopping when you are hungry. Hunger can lead to quick, reckless choices and over-buying. Shopping without a list can yield the same results, so don't shop without your list in hand.

We're now ready to navigate the aisles of a store. Let's go on a virtual grocery trip together, and I'll give you aisle-by-aisle shopping pointers.

Fresh Produce

- Start here by filling your cart with a colorful variety of fresh produce.
- Check produce sales and buy in season when possible.
- If you're not sure which apples or peaches are tastiest, ask the grocer. Many will even wash and cut a piece of fruit for you to taste.
- If you buy a bulk amount of a fresh fruit or vegetable that doesn't taste good, don't hesitate to return the rest and get your money back.

Grains/Breads, Cereals, Pasta, and Rice

- Choose whole-grain versions with 5 or more grams of fiber per serving, if available.

Dressings, Sauces, and Condiments

- Choose low-fat or light versions with high flavor, such as salsa, light vinaigrette salad dressing, balsamic vinegar, spicy mustard, prepared spaghetti or light teriyaki sauce, sandwich pickle slices, and bottled peppers.
- Meat marinades are popular but remember that they don't have to be just for meat. You can use Thai, jerk-style, and sweet and sour marinades on roasted vegetables for a change of pace.
- Choose heart healthy cooking oils like canola oil and olive oil.

Canned Goods

- Choose a variety of canned beans, bean soups, water-packed tuna, and other salad toppings such as hearts of palm and artichoke hearts.
- Choose low-fat or fat-free chicken broth, vegetable broth, and canned tomatoes. Look for reduced-sodium versions.

> ### ⋙ *Nibble on This* ⋘
> New research shows that low-fat dairy product consumption may enhance weight loss.

Dairy/Milk, Yogurt, and Cheeses

- Choose low-fat or fat-free versions.
- Try cholesterol-free, commercial egg substitutes, and egg whites, sold in cartons.
- Low-fat cottage cheese can be an excellent snack with some sliced fresh fruit.
- Light string cheese is an easy preportioned snack.
- Try Light Laughing Cow cheese for a low-calorie, great-tasting spread.
- Instead of stick butter and margarine, choose light tub margarine like Brummel & Brown or liquid margarine.
- Yogurt has naturally occurring milk sugars, but look for yogurts with less added sugar. Try adding whole fruits to plain yogurt or try the "lite" varieties.

Other Protein

- Choose lean turkey slices, skinless chicken/rotisserie chicken, salmon, or other fresh fish/crab/shrimp, fresh soy products (refrigerated in the produce section), and less red meat and pork products.
- Select reduced-fat peanut butter and buy small bags of nuts or soy nuts to keep on hand for sprinkling on salads and stir-frys.

- Try dried beans and packaged bean soups, many of which can be made in minutes. (If a higher-fiber diet is new to you and your body is taking time to adjust, stop by the antacid aisle for an antigas product, like Bean-O).
- Vegetarian chili can add a burst of flavor to soy hot dogs, turkey burgers, and potatoes.

Freezer

- Select bags of frozen fruits and vegetables that allow you to use only what you need.
- Choose frozen soy products like Boca Burgers and Boca Crumbles (for sloppy joes and chili).
- Bags of frozen shrimp or scallops make great last-minute stir-fry dishes.
- Check for frozen salmon and other fish. Some retailers offer it frozen for a fraction of the fresh price.
- Look for frozen desserts such as fruit juice bars, fat-free fudge bars, and fat-free or light yogurt.
- Try calorie-controlled Healthy Choice, Lean Cuisine, or Weight Watchers Smart Ones meals. Remember, you can add frozen vegetables to these frozen meals to make them more nutritious and filling.

Seasonings

- Choose salt-free herb and pepper blends like Mrs. Dash. Try specialty Cajun, Creole, Thai, and Italian seasonings or McCormick Grill Mates.
- Try seasonings like cumin, curry, herbs de Provence, hot chili powder, crushed red pepper flakes, rosemary, and thyme to add more kick to your cooking.
- Keep empty spice jars and refill them with bulk spices. Buying self-serve spices by weight saves money and it allows you to purchase in smaller quantities so that you're cooking with fresher, more flavorful spices.

Health Foods

- Check labels, as all products in this section are not always healthy. For example, some granola cereals are high in fat and calories.

If the grocery store doesn't have a certain product, you can ask them to carry it. And save yourself time. If a super recipe ingredient sounds uncommon (like whole wheat lasagna noodles, quinoa, or bok choy), I recommend that you call the supermarket first and ask if and where they carry it.

Use Healthy Kitchen Tools

The following tools allow you to cook healthier and more efficiently:

- two good nonstick pans (one wok and one nonstick pan is fine also) along with wooden spoons (for stir-frying or sautéing)
- indoor electric grill (to cook chicken, fish, lean meats, and vegetables)
- grilling tray and basket (to cook chicken, fish, lean meats, and vegetables on outdoor grills)
- oil spray canister or use commercial nonstick cooking spray (uses less oil than with a brush)
- steamer basket (for steaming vegetables)
- colander (for rinsing canned beans and vegetables—reduces sodium levels)
- roasting pans (for roasting vegetables, including potatoes)
- food processor, blender, or hand mixer (for making dips and thickening soups)
- microwave (for quickly cooking veggies, popping popcorn, and reheating healthy leftovers)
- kitchen shears (for cutting fresh herbs and trimming any visible fat from meat)
- measuring cups, spoons, and kitchen scale (for following healthy recipes)

Save Prep Time

A couple of minutes saved here and a couple saved there can really add up. I recommend that you try these time-saving tips:

- Use minced garlic in a jar instead of fresh garlic (found in the produce section).
- Use frozen vegetables and fruits when indicated in the recipe or when you have them on hand.

- Buy fresh fruits and vegetables already cut up and ready to go (such as cubed pineapple, cut-up lettuce, sliced mushrooms).
- Check the grocer's salad bar for precut fruits and vegetables.
- Use refrigerated or frozen already cooked chicken strips for salads or stir-frys (though the sodium content is often quite high in these products). A healthier option is to grill and slice chicken breasts on the weekend and freeze in portion-controlled freezer bags.
- Use canned chicken or vegetable broth instead of making your own. Look for reduced-sodium versions.
- Use canned beans instead of the dried varieties. Be sure to rinse and drain them to reduce the sodium content.

Make Meals in Minutes

Registered dietitian Amy Baltes tells patients always to have on hand the ingredients to make five quick and easy meals. Convenience items make this task easier than it has ever been. Here are some ideas:

- Frozen veggie burger, whole wheat bun, vegetarian baked beans, and vegetable.
- Whole wheat pasta with ready-made pasta sauce and a salad.
- Black bean burritos (spread whole-grain tortilla with warm, canned beans, salsa, low-fat cheese, tomatoes, and lettuce. Roll and serve).
- Vegetarian pizza (top ready-made pizza crust with pizza sauce, low-fat mozzarella cheese, and presliced mushrooms; cook according to package directions).
- Canned soup served with entrée salad made with bagged lettuce and veggies, and topped with low-fat tuna salad (made with water-packed tuna, white beans drained and rinsed, chopped green onion, light mayonnaise) and light vinaigrette dressing.

I also recommend that you think about the healthier take-out meals in your neighborhood that can be ordered in minutes. Consider vegetarian pizza with only a sprinkle of cheese, veggie baked potato with salad and light dressing, vegetarian or turkey sub sandwich without mayonnaise, bean soup with whole-grain bagel and hummus, or vegetarian Asian dishes that are not deep fried and are light on the oil. Making healthy requests "to go" can save you hundreds upon hundreds of calories.

Doctor Up

"Doctoring up" is an important healthy cooking skill that I recommend you practice and refine. Use condiments, herbs, and seasonings to boost the flavor of your new healthy meals. Here are some examples of doctoring up the above meals in minutes.

- Add grilled onions, sliced tomatoes, and barbecue sauce to awaken the flavor of veggie burgers.
- Add ground turkey or frozen veggie crumbles, frozen bell peppers, and grated parmesan cheese to make a heartier pasta dish.
- Season beans for burritos with hot sauce and chili powder to make them spicier.
- Add soy pepperoni and crushed red pepper to enhance the flavor of vegetarian pizza.
- Add grated parmesan cheese to canned soup and garlic powder and dried cranberries to your entrée salad.
- Add low-fat chunky salsa and 1 cup Boca Burger crumbles to a can of black beans for a fast and zesty chili.

Doctor Down

"Doctoring down" is another healthy cooking skill whereby you lower the calorie and fat contents of your favorite recipes. Here are some common doctoring down strategies that I recommend you try:

- Instead of regular cheeses, sour cream, or mayo, use reduced-fat cheeses, low-fat sour cream, and light mayo.
- Instead of heavy cream, use nonfat milk or evaporated skim milk.
- Instead of 1 whole egg, use 2 egg whites or commercial egg substitutes.
- Instead of sautéing in butter or margarine, sauté in olive oil or canola oil, or use nonstick cooking spray with vegetable or chicken broth.
- Remove the skin from poultry and visible fat from meats.
- Experiment with cutting the sugar in some recipes by a third to a half.

■ Experiment with cutting the fat in some recipes by a third to a half. When baking, try replacing butter with more heart-healthy fats such as canola oil.

■ Use commercial fat-free, fruit-based butter and oil replacement for baking (in jars near the cooking oils).

Batch Cook

Usually done when you have more time, like on the weekend, cooking in large batches and then freezing portions allows you to enjoy healthy foods during your busy workweek. Using different-sized freezer containers converts leftovers into meals that you can enjoy in minutes. Label the containers with the contents and date frozen. If you excavate chili dated last year, throw it out.

Avoid Nutrition Amnesia

Our super food recipe nutritionist has observed that consumers often become lax about the amount of fat they use during cooking. For example, if you tend to eyeball the amount of oil during cooking, you can easily be doubling or tripling the recommended quantity called for in a healthy recipe. Sticking with measured recipe amounts will help you reduce your calorie intake and, ultimately, the pounds on the scale.

Overcome the Short-Order-Cook Syndrome

If some of your family members are resistant to eating healthier meals, don't be surprised if you start feeling like a short-order cook. To overcome this common syndrome, try the following strategies:

■ Talk seriously with family members about your health goals.

■ Remind yourself that healthy cooking does not mean giving up all of your favorite recipes. By making just a few ingredient substitutions (doctoring down) and always adding extra vegetables and salads on the side, old favorites can become healthy new favorites.

■ Use the "let's make a deal" strategy. For example, if they agree to sample healthier meals two times a week to start and without complaining, you agree to still prepare some of their favorite dishes on other days of the week. Or if they agree to sample healthier meals, you agree to "doctor up" their portions just the way they like them.

■ If your family regularly eats higher-calorie and -fat entrees, you can enjoy their "sides" (such as bean or vegetable soups, large salads, roasted vegetables, whole-grain breads, bean salads, and fresh fruit) as your entrées. Also keep frozen healthy meals on standby in the freezer.

Super Recipe Basics

The following thirty super recipes were created by Eileen Vincent, MS, RD, LD, with eye appeal, good taste, portion control, and your nutrition in mind. Each recipe features at least one super food (indicated with a ✸ symbol) and several other nutritious plant-based ingredients. By definition, super foods are exclusively of plant origin, which inherently contain "super" dietary sources of at least one vitamin or mineral or dietary fiber ("super" source = 20 percent or more of Daily Reference Intake for a particular nutrient). Though recipes may contain sources of other nutrients, only the "super" source nutrients are highlighted at the bottom of each Nutrition Facts label. These nutrients may reduce your risks of heart disease, certain cancers, and diabetes as well as improve bone density, lower blood cholesterol, and boost your overall immunity. See the tables at the end of this chapter for more information on the nutrients and health benefits of eating a diet rich in super foods.

All recipes have been carefully balanced for the right amount of nutrients and calories and were analyzed using a research-nutrient database (University of Minnesota, Nutrition Coordinating Center Nutrition Data System, Version 2.93). Since the entrée is usually the greatest contributor of fat and calories for lunch or dinner, one serving of either a super meaty main event or a super meatless recipe provides fewer than 325 calories and 10 grams of total fat (per recipe; see nutrition facts). The sample menu that corresponds with each super food recipe illustrates how that recipe can fit into a healthy lunch or dinner containing fewer than 650 calories total. You can use the recommended serving sizes listed on the recipe as well as the standard serving sizes on page 40 as calorie- and portion-control guides.

Each super food recipe is a creative combination of mostly plant-based ingredients that render tasty dishes for you to enjoy. Instead of using fat as a flavor enhancer, the super food recipes call for either fresh or minimally processed plant-based ingredients, herbs, and spices to maximize the flavor and nutritional value of each dish. Additionally, time-crunched dieters will like the multiple portions yielded by most recipes; you can divide the leftovers into recommended portions and stow them in the freezer for a healthy meal on the run.

I encourage you to try these super recipes in your own kitchen. Some of you may want to follow each recipe exactly, while others may be more adventurous by adding your favorite seasonings or substituting another ingredient that you happen to have on hand. Putting your own spin on a super food recipe is an easy way to develop your own healthy cooking style—as you also increase your and your family's enjoyment. Besides, isn't that what home cooking's all about? Bon appétit!

📑 *This symbol denotes that a sample menu recipe is included.*

Super Starts

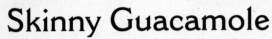

Skinny Guacamole

Asparagus serves as a low-fat substitute for avocados in this alternative guacamole recipe.

Ingredients

★ *2 packages (9 ounces each) unseasoned frozen asparagus (no sauce added), defrosted or 1 pound fresh asparagus, steamed, cut*
¼ cup fresh cilantro, finely chopped
2 tablespoons lime juice
4 tablespoons low-fat mayonnaise
2 tablespoons water
½ cup onion, finely chopped
3 tablespoons garlic, minced
★ *1 can (15 ounces) diced tomatoes, drained well, or 1½ cups fresh tomatoes, peeled*
½ teaspoon salt or garlic salt (or to taste)
4 drops hot pepper sauce (or to taste)

Directions
1. Puree asparagus and cilantro in blender. Add lime juice, low-fat mayo, and 2 tablespoons of water or more as necessary to reach a thick, smooth consistency.
2. In a medium-size bowl, combine pureed asparagus with onion, garlic, tomatoes, salt, and hot pepper sauce.
3. Chill for at least an hour before serving.
4. Serve with raw jicama slices, baby carrots, red bell pepper slices, baked tortilla chips, or garlic-flavored melba toast.

Sample Menu

Skinny Guacamole 🗹
Served with raw vegetables and
baked tortilla chips
Barley Chicken Chili 🗹
Low-fat sandwich cookies

NUTRITION FACTS

Serving size ¼ cup
Servings per recipe 8

Amount per serving
Calories 59   Calories from fat 27

Total Fat	1 gram
Saturated Fat	0 grams
Cholesterol	0 milligrams
Sodium	286 milligrams
Total Carbohydrate	8 grams
Dietary Fiber	2 grams
Sugars	2 grams
Protein	2.5 grams
Super nutrients: vitamin C and folate	

Broiled Vegetables

The intense heat from broiling "sweetens" the flavor of this colorful vegetable dish.

Ingredients

Nonstick cooking spray

I large red onion, peeled and sliced

⭐ *2 large red, yellow, or green bell peppers, cored and sliced in strips*

I large eggplant (about I pound), thinly cut crosswise with peel in 1/8" slices

I large zucchini, cut lengthwise into 3"-long strips

I pound fresh green beans (3 1/2 cups), ends snipped off

1/3 cup reduced-fat Italian or red wine vinegar dressing (no more than 5 grams fat/2 tablespoons, per label)

2 tablespoons chopped garlic

Garlic or onion salt to taste

Directions

1. Turn broiler on high. Arrange oven rack on level closest to broiler heat.
2. Line cookie sheet or broiling pan with foil. Grease foil with a thin coat of cooking spray.
3. Place onion and pepper slices on the cookie sheet. Spray vegetables well with cooking spray.
4. Broil for 10–15 minutes or until vegetables turn golden brown. Turn vegetables over, spray with a light coat of cooking spray, and broil until backside is golden brown. Transfer vegetables to a serving dish.
5. Roast eggplant slices, zucchini, and green beans *separately* as indicated in steps 3–4 (each vegetable has its own cooking time). Add to serving dish.
6. Season vegetables with salad dressing, chopped garlic, and salt.
7. Chill for at least 1 hour (preferably marinate overnight). Dish peaks in flavor a day after preparation. Serve cold or at room temperature.

<u>Sample</u> <u>Menu</u>

Broiled Vegetables ☐
Tex-Mex Stuffed Sweet Potato ☐
Baked whole-grain crackers
Lady fingers

NUTRITION FACTS

Serving size 1 cup
Servings per recipe 8

Amount per serving

Calories 95   Calories from fat 36

Total Fat	4 grams
Saturated Fat	0.5 grams
Cholesterol	0 milligrams
Sodium	179 milligrams
Total Carbohydrate	14 grams
Dietary Fiber	4 grams
Sugars	5 grams
Protein	3 grams
Super nutrients: vitamins A and C	

Mini-Veggie Wraps

This "appeteaser" features a creative use of hummus, a flavorful garbanzo bean dip.

Ingredients

Tortillas:
6 (8" diameter) flour tortillas (less than 3 grams total fat per tortilla as indicated on label)
Tip: Recommend using spinach, sun-dried tomato, or whole wheat tortillas.

Hummus:
Nonfat cooking spray
★ *2 medium red bell peppers, cored and sliced into strips*
★ *15-ounce can garbanzo beans, drained*
¼ cup water
1 tablespoon garlic
1 tablespoon sesame seed oil or tahini paste
1 tablespoon lemon juice
⅛ teaspoon salt (or to taste)

Vegetables:
★ *¾ cup raw broccoli flowerets, chopped*
★ *½ cup raw carrots, grated*
½ cup green onion, chopped
2 tablespoons black olives, finely chopped (optional)

Directions

1. Line a cookie sheet with foil and spray with nonfat cooking spray. Place red pepper slices on cookie sheet.
2. Broil peppers for about 10 minutes or until dark brown around the edges.

3. Puree garbanzo beans and water in a blender.

4. Add cooled peppers and remaining ingredients for hummus to blender. Puree until mixture reaches a grainy, puddinglike consistency. If necessary, add 1 or more tablespoons of additional water to reach desired consistency.

5. Spread ⅓ cup hummus on each tortilla, especially along the edges.

6. Sprinkle each tortilla with:
   ❖ 2 tablespoons broccoli
   ❖ 1 tablespoon each of grated carrots and green onion
   ❖ 1 teaspoon chopped olives

7. Wrap vegetable-filled tortilla into a roll. Spread a small bit of additional hummus around the edges to help seal the tortilla.

8. Refrigerate tortillas at least 1 hour. Slice into 2"-long pieces (each tortilla makes 4 slices).

NUTRITION FACTS	
Serving size 2 (2"-long wraps)	
Servings per recipe 12	
Amount per serving	
Calories 151	Calories from fat 36
Total Fat	4 grams
Saturated fat	0.5 gram
Cholesterol	0 milligrams
Sodium	218 milligrams
Total Carbohydrate	24 grams
Dietary Fiber	4 grams
Sugars	2 grams
Protein	5.5 grams
Super nutrients: vitamins A and C, folate	

Sample Menu

Mini-Veggie Wraps 🥡
Hearty Barley Lentil Chowder 🥡
Mixed green salad with nonfat or light dressing
Nonfat chocolate pudding
Garnished with vanilla wafers

Super Soups

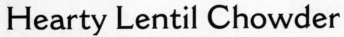

Hearty Lentil Chowder

The barley and lentils are so filling in this soup that it can serve as a main course for a light meal.

Ingredients

★ *1 cup dried red lentils (can substitute brown lentils)*

1 large yellow or white onion, finely chopped

3 tablespoons garlic, minced

2 cups celery (4 large stalks), finely chopped

1 tablespoon canola oil or olive oil

2/3 cup dried pearled or Scotch barley (not quick-cooking barley)

★ *2 cans (15 ounces each) diced tomatoes with liquid*

★ *1 cup diced carrots*

★ *1 cup parsley, finely chopped*

4 cups nonfat chicken or vegetable broth

2 cups water

1/2 teaspoon salt (or to taste)

1/2 teaspoon dried thyme

1 teaspoon dried basil

1 teaspoon dried oregano

1/4 teaspoon black pepper

Directions

1. Line a colander with paper towel. Pour dry lentils on top and rinse well. Transfer lentils into a soup pot.
2. Brown chopped onion, garlic, and celery with oil in a small frying pan. Transfer vegetables to soup pot.
3. Add remaining ingredients and seasonings to the soup pot. Cook over medium heat until soup mixture boils.

4. Lower heat to low and simmer for 1 to 1½ hours, or until both barley and lentils are tender. Since soup will thicken when it cools, you may want to add water when you reheat.

5. Soup can be stored in the refrigerator for several days or frozen in portion-size containers.

NUTRITION FACTS

Serving size 1 cup
Servings per recipe 12

Amount per serving	
Calories 138	Calories from fat 9

Total Fat	1 gram
Saturated Fat	0 grams
Cholesterol	0 milligrams
Sodium	593 milligrams
Total Carbohydrate	26 grams
Dietary Fiber	7 grams
Sugars	2 grams
Protein	8 grams

Super nutrients: vitamins A and C, folate; potassium

Sample Menu

Mini-Veggie Wraps ☐
Hearty Lentil Chowder ☐
Mixed greens salad with nonfat or light dressing
Nonfat chocolate pudding
Garnished with vanilla wafers

Moroccan Pumpkin Soup

Savor the unique flavor combination of pumpkin, black beans, tomatoes, and seasonings in this quick-and-easy soup.

Ingredients

1 large red onion, finely chopped

2 tablespoons minced garlic

1 tablespoon canola oil or olive oil

★ 2 cans (15 ounces each) diced tomatoes with liquid

★ 1 can (15 ounces) unsweetened mashed pumpkin

★ 3 cans (15 ounces each) black beans with liquid

1 cup nonfat chicken broth

¼ cup cooking sherry

2 tablespoons seasoned rice vinegar (can substitute apple cider vinegar plus

   ⅓ teaspoon salt)

1 tablespoon + 2 teaspoons ground cumin

½ teaspoon salt (or to taste)

½ teaspoon ground cinnamon

¼ teaspoon cayenne pepper

Nonstick cooking spray

Directions

1. Sauté onion and garlic with oil in a small frying pan.
2. In a large soup pan, combine the onion and garlic with remaining ingredients. Cook over medium heat until soup mixture boils.
3. Lower heat to low and simmer the soup for approximately 15 minutes. Since soup will thicken when it cools, you may want to add water when you reheat.
4. Soup can be stored in the refrigerator for several days or frozen in portion-size containers. Soup peaks in flavor a day after preparation.

<u>Sample</u> <u>Menu</u>

Moroccan Pumpkin Soup ☐
Grilled chicken breast
Asian Sesame Salad Greens ☐
Served with garlic-flavored melba toast
Frozen fruit juice bar

NUTRITION FACTS

Serving size 1 cup
Servings per recipe 10

Amount per serving
Calories 244   Calories from fat 23

Total Fat	2.5 grams
Saturated Fat	0.5 grams
Cholesterol	0 milligrams
Sodium	850 milligrams
Total Carbohydrate	44 grams
Dietary Fiber	11 grams
Sugars	6 grams
Protein	13 grams

Super nutrients: vitamins A and C,
folate; iron, potassium

Chunky Butternut Squash Soup

Cutting the butternut squash requires a little effort. But the reward is the wonderful color, taste, and texture that this unusual vegetable provides.

Ingredients

★ 6 cups raw butternut squash, cubed (about 1 medium squash)

1 cup celery (4 medium stalks), diced

1 large yellow onion, chopped

4 tablespoons chopped garlic

1 tablespoon canola oil or olive oil

2 cans (15 ounces each) nonfat chicken or vegetable broth

★ 1 can (15 ounces) canellini (white kidney) beans, drained

★ 1 cup fresh parsley, finely chopped

2 tablespoons white cooking wine

1 tablespoon dark brown sugar

1½ teaspoons fresh or ground ginger

2 teaspoons ground cumin

¼ teaspoon salt (or to taste)

¼ teaspoon black pepper

Directions

1. Cut squash in half crosswise. Remove peel by cutting outer layer lengthwise with a *very* sharp knife. Remove seeds and cut peeled squash in ½-inch cubes.
2. Steam cubed squash for 12 minutes or until tender.
3. Sauté celery, onions, and garlic in oil.
4. Combine cooked squash and sautéed vegetables in a medium-size soup pot.
5. Add broth, beans, parsley, wine, sugar, and seasonings.
6. Cook over medium heat, stirring constantly, for 15 minutes, or until soup begins to boil.

<u>Sample</u> <u>Menu</u>

Chunky Butternut Squash Soup 🗹
Baked rainbow trout
Seasoned with fresh herbs
Sautéed spinach
Crusty whole-grain roll
Fig bars

NUTRITION FACTS

Serving size 1 cup
Servings per recipe 12

Amount per serving
Calories 125   Calories from fat 18

Total Fat	2 grams
Saturated Fat	0 grams
Cholesterol	0 milligrams
Sodium	470 milligrams
Total Carbohydrate	23 grams
Dietary Fiber	4 grams
Sugars	4 grams
Protein	6 grams

Super nutrients: vitamins A and C,
folate; potassium

Super Meatless

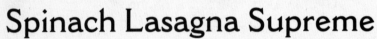

Spinach Lasagna Supreme

This restaurant-quality vegetarian lasagna will delight even meat lovers in your family.

Ingredients

Nonstick cooking spray

8-ounce package whole wheat lasagna, uncooked (can substitute regular lasagna noodles)

8 ounces fresh mushrooms, sliced (optional)

4 tablespoons minced garlic

1 tablespoon canola oil or olive oil

★ 16-ounce package chopped frozen spinach, thawed, drained well

32 ounces fat-free ricotta cheese

½ teaspoon salt (or to taste)

26 ounces meatless spaghetti sauce (commercial sauce providing no more than 4 grams fat / ½ cup per nutrition label)

2 cups grated part-skim mozzarella cheese

½ cup grated parmesan cheese

Directions

1. Spray a 13" × 9" lasagna pan with nonstick cooking spray.
2. Line the bottom of the pan with uncooked lasagna noodles.
3. Sauté mushrooms and garlic with oil in a small frying pan.
4. Mix together sautéed mushrooms and garlic with ricotta, spinach, and salt in a large bowl.
5. Spread half of spinach and ricotta mixture with a spatula on the bottom layer of lasagna noodles.
6. Top with half of spaghetti sauce.
7. Sprinkle 1 cup mozzarella and ¼ cup parmesan on top of the spaghetti sauce layer.
8. Place another layer of uncooked lasagna noodles on top of the cheeses.

9. Repeat steps 5–7 to create second lasagna layer.
10. DO NOT cover the second layer with lasagna noodles. Otherwise the lasagna will be dry after baking.
11. Cover pan with foil and bake at 350° for 1 hour. Remove foil for the last 5–10 minutes of baking to brown the cheese.
12. Let stand for 10 minutes before cutting into 16 squares.

NUTRITION FACTS

Serving size 1 square
Servings per recipe 16

Amount per serving
Calories 217   Calories from fat 45

Total Fat	5 grams
Saturated Fat	2 grams
Cholesterol	10 milligrams
Sodium	579 milligrams
Total Carbohydrate	28 grams
Dietary Fiber	3 grams
Sugars	5 grams
Protein	17 grams

Super nutrients: vitamins A and C; bonus from cheeses: 297 milligrams calcium

Sample Menu

Tossed green salad with seasoned rice wine vinegar
Spinach Lasagna Supreme
Garlic bread made with light tub margarine
Apricot Bars

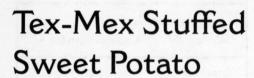

Tex-Mex Stuffed Sweet Potato

A homemade BBQ sauce adds lots of zest to these sweet potato fixin's.

Ingredients

★ *3 medium sweet potatoes*
★ *I cup canned black beans, drained*
⅓ cup catsup
★ *I tablespoon blackstrap or dark molasses*
I tablespoon minced garlic
I tablespoon chili powder
Dash cayenne pepper (optional)

Directions

1. Wrap each sweet potato in a moist paper towel. Microwave potatoes individually on high until soft in the middle. Or bake potatoes (no paper towel) in conventional oven at 400° for 45 minutes.
2. Combine remaining ingredients in a saucepan. Cook until mixture just starts to boil.
3. Halve each cooked sweet potato lengthwise. Top each potato with ⅓ of black bean mixture.

<u>Sample</u> <u>Menu</u>

Broiled Vegetables ☑
Tex-Mex Sweet Potato ☑
Baked whole-grain crackers
Lady fingers

NUTRITION FACTS

Serving size 1 potato
Servings per recipe 3

Amount per serving
Calories 246   Calories from fat 5

Total Fat	0.5 grams
Saturated Fat	0 grams
Cholesterol	0 milligrams
Sodium	549 milligrams
Total Carbohydrate	55 grams
Dietary Fiber	7 grams
Sugars	17 grams
Protein	8 grams

Super nutrients: vitamins A, B_6, and C, folate; potassium

Eggplant et Cetera Parmesan

Downsizing portions of cheese and oil provides a lighter version of a traditional Italian recipe.

Ingredients

*1 medium eggplant **with** skin, cut into ⅛" round inch slices*

Nonstick cooking spray

★ *1 cup dry TVP (textured vegetable protein), optional with 1 cup boiled water*

2½ cups meatless spaghetti sauce (commercial sauce providing no more than 4 grams fat / ½ cup per nutrition label)

★ *1 medium red pepper, cored and diced*

2 cups mushrooms, chopped

2 tablespoons minced garlic

¾ cup grated part-skim mozzarella cheese

⅓ cup grated parmesan cheese

Salt and pepper to taste

Directions

1. Line a cookie sheet with foil. Place eggplant slices on the cookie sheet and spray with nonstick cooking spray. Broil on high for 5 minutes or until eggplant is golden brown.
2. Lower oven to 375°.
3. Spray an 11" × 7" Pyrex baking dish with nonstick cooking spray.
4. Mix 1 cup boiled water with 1 cup TVP. Let sit for 15 minutes.

NUTRITION FACTS	
Serving size 1½ cups	
Servings per recipe 4	
Amount per serving (with TVP)	
Calories 311	Calories from fat 81
Total Fat	9 grams
Saturated Fat	4 grams
Cholesterol	16 milligrams
Sodium	901 milligrams
Total Carbohydrate	40 grams
Dietary Fiber	8 grams
Sugars	11 grams
Protein	23 grams
Super nutrients: vitamins A, B_6, and C, potassium; bonus from cheeses and TVP: 330 milligrams calcium	

5. Mix together rehydrated TVP with spaghetti sauce.

6. Sauté red pepper, mushrooms, and garlic with cooking spray.

7. Layer half the eggplant slices, red pepper, mushrooms, and garlic in the Pyrex dish. Season with salt and pepper as desired.

8. Top vegetables with half of TVP/spaghetti sauce mixture (or just spaghetti sauce), then mozzarella and parmesan cheeses.

9. Repeat steps 7 and 8 to create second layer.

10. Cover pan with foil and bake at 350° for 45 minutes. Remove foil for last 5–10 minutes to allow cheese to brown.

11. Let stand for 10 minutes before serving. Garnish with 1 tablespoon of parmesan cheese sprinkled on top.

NUTRITION FACTS	
Serving size 1¼ cups	
Servings per recipe 4	
Amount per serving (no TVP)	
Calories 272	Calories from fat 81
Total Fat	9 grams
Saturated Fat	4 grams
Cholesterol	18 milligrams
Sodium	894 milligrams
Total Carbohydrate	38 grams
Dietary Fiber	7 grams
Sugars	10 grams
Protein	14 grams
Super nutrients: vitamins A, B_6, and C, potassium; bonus from cheeses and TVP: 330 milligrams calcium	

Sample Menu

Tossed green salad with seasoned red wine vinegar

Eggplant et Cetera Parmesan ▱

Served on a bed of whole wheat pasta

Kale 'n' Mushrooms ▱

Low-fat lemon cookies

Super Veggie Patty

This is the ultimate meatless burger packed with beans, oats, and five different types of vegetables.

Ingredients

1 medium onion, finely chopped
1 cup fresh mushrooms, sliced
★ *1 cup red bell pepper, chopped*
1 tablespoon canola oil or olive oil
★ *1 can (15 ounces) pinto beans, drained*
1 cup grated zucchini (about one small zucchini)
★ *1 cup chopped raw broccoli*
1 cup grated light mozzarella cheese (less than 4 grams fat per ¼ cup)
2 egg whites, lightly whipped
1 cup dry oats
2 tablespoons minced garlic
3 tablespoons fresh basil, chopped (or 1 tablespoon dried)
½ teaspoon ground marjoram
½ teaspoon ground thyme
½ teaspoon salt or garlic salt
½ teaspoon black pepper
Nonstick cooking spray
Low-fat spaghetti sauce, catsup, or barbecue sauce (optional)

Directions

1. Sauté onion, mushrooms, and red pepper in oil.
2. In a medium-size mixing bowl, mash pinto beans with a fork.
3. Add onion mixture and remaining ingredients (except cooking spray and optional sauces) to the beans. Mix well.
4. Refrigerate mixture at least 15 minutes.

5. Pat about ¾ cup of mixture with hands to form 6 patties (approximately 4" diameter and ¾" thick).

6. Place patties on a broiler pan, lined with foil that is greased with nonfat cooking spray.

7. Broil patties on low for 10 minutes or until golden brown.

8. Carefully flip over patties and broil for an additional 10 minutes.

9. Serve hot with 2 tablespoons of low-fat spaghetti sauce (warmed), catsup, or barbecue sauce.

Note: Uncooked patties will keep, covered, for 3 days in the refrigerator.

NUTRITION FACTS

Serving size 1 patty
Servings per recipe 6

Amount per serving 6	
Calories 256	Calories from fat 54

Total Fat	6 grams
Saturated Fat	2 grams
Cholesterol	37 milligrams
Sodium	436 milligrams
Total Carbohydrate	29 grams
Dietary Fiber	9 grams
Sugars	3 grams
Protein	16 grams

Super nutrients: vitamins A and C, calcium

Sample Menu

Roasted sweet potato wedges
Super Veggie Patty
Garnished with 2 tablespoons marinara sauce
Angel food cake
Garnished with fresh strawberries and
nonfat vanilla yogurt

Cruciferous Veggie Casserole

Can't remember the last time that you ate Brussels sprouts?
Two members of the cruciferous vegetable family are nestled in this dish.

Ingredients

Cheese Sauce:

3 tablespoons flour

¼ cup water

2 tablespoons light tub margarine (no more than 5 grams fat/tablespoon per label)

12-ounce can evaporated nonfat milk

1 cup grated Jarlsberg light Swiss or light cheddar cheese (no more than 4 grams
    fat/ounce per label)

2 tablespoons cooking sherry

½ teaspoon salt (or to taste)

½ teaspoon dry mustard

⅛ teaspoon white pepper

Casserole:

1 cup raw mushrooms, sliced

1 medium onion, finely chopped

Nonstick cooking spray

★ 2 cups cauliflower, chopped (can use fresh or frozen, thawed)

★ 2 cups (about 12) sliced Brussels sprouts (fresh or frozen, thawed)

1 cup cooked (½ cup dry) wild rice (can substitute a brown and wild rice blend)

★ ¼ cup parsley, finely chopped

Directions

1. Dissolve flour in water.
2. Melt margarine in a medium-size sauce pan. Add flour mixture.
3. Carefully add evaporated milk. Whisk well until flour dissolves.

4. Cook sauce over low-medium heat until it begins to thicken (stir sauce often with wire whisk to avoid burning on the bottom of the pan).

5. Add cheese, sherry, and seasonings to thickened sauce.

6. Continue to cook sauce over low-medium heat until mixture begins to boil. Remove sauce from heat.

7. Sauté mushrooms and onions using cooking spray until golden brown.

8. In a large mixing bowl, combine sautéed mushrooms and onions with cauliflower, Brussels sprouts, and cooked rice.

9. Add thickened cheese sauce to vegetable/rice mixture. Mix well.

10. Pour casserole mixture into a 2-quart casserole dish, sprayed with nonstick cooking spray. Garnish with chopped parsley.

11. Cover and bake at 375° for 30 minutes. Remove cover during the last 5 minutes of baking for a golden brown crust.

NUTRITION FACTS	
Serving size 1¼ cups	
Servings per recipe 6	
Amount per serving	
Calories 308	Calories from fat 72
Total Fat	8 grams
Saturated Fat	3.5 grams
Cholestrol	18 milligrams
Sodium	632 milligrams
Total Carbohydrate	38 grams
Dietary Fiber	6 grams
Sugars	2 grams
Protein	22 grams
Super nutrients: vitamins A, B$_6$, and C, folate, potassium; bonus from dairy: 520 milligrams calcium	

Sample Menu

Garden salad with light dressing
Cruciferous Veggie Casserole ☐
Pumpernickel roll
Two-Berry Crisp ☐

Baked Swiss Chard Frittata

A favorite Spanish dish with a healthier twist.
Swiss chard adds a distinctive flavor to this heart-smart vegetable omelet.

Ingredients

1 small white potato, peeled, thinly sliced using a kitchen grater or food processor

1/2 cup onion, finely chopped

✭ *1 cup red bell pepper, cored and chopped*

2 tablespoons chopped garlic

Nonstick cooking spray

✭ *3 cups Swiss chard, chopped; use dark green leaves that are removed from white midrib stalks (can substitute 3 cups fresh spinach)*

1 cup commercial egg substitute (can substitute 8 egg whites, but flavor is compromised)

1/4 cup skim milk

1 cup grated Jarlsberg light Swiss or other light cheese (no more than 4 grams fat/ounce per label)

1/4 teaspoon salt

1/8 teaspoon cayenne or white pepper

Directions

1. Brown potato, onion, pepper, and garlic in a large skillet using nonstick cooking spray.
2. Microwave Swiss chard on high for 1 minute or until leaves wilt.
3. Beat egg substitute with milk until frothy. Add grated cheese and seasonings. Mix well.
4. Spray an 8-inch ovenproof ceramic or glass dish with nonstick cooking spray.
5. Evenly spread cooked chard, potato, and onions in baking dish. Pour egg mixture over vegetables.

6. Bake uncovered at 350° for about 45 minutes or until egg mixture is firm (test doneness using a toothpick or knife) and top is golden brown.
7. Immediately after baking, run a knife along the sides of the dish for easier removal.

NUTRITION FACTS

Serving size ½ omelet
Servings per recipe 2

Amount per serving	
Calories 310	Calories from fat 90

Total Fat	10 grams
Saturated Fat	6 grams
Cholesterol	30 milligrams
Sodium	845 milligrams
Total Carbohydrate	28 grams
Dietary Fiber	4 grams
Sugars	5 grams
Protein	30 grams

Super nutrients: vitamins A, B_6, and C, iron, magnesium, potassium; bonus from dairy: 528 milligrams calcium

Sample Menu

Swiss Chard Frittata ☑
California Jicama Salad ☑
Crusty whole wheat roll
Fat-free raspberry bars

Polynesian Stir-Fry

Molasses is a "black" goldmine of nutrition because it is rich in iron, calcium, and other minerals. This dark syrup provides a robust flavor to a meatless stir-fry.

Ingredients

Sauce:

3 tablespoons cornstarch

¼ cup cold water

★ ¼ cup blackstrap or dark molasses

½ cup chicken or vegetable broth

2 tablespoons chopped garlic

★ 2 tablespoons sunflower seeds

1 teaspoon minced fresh garlic

2 tablespoons lite (reduced-sodium) soy sauce (or to taste)

⅛ teaspoon cayenne pepper (or to taste)

1 tablespoon granulated sugar

Vegetable Mixture:

1 tablespoon sesame seed oil

★ 2 cups baby carrots, sliced, lengthwise

★ 2 cups broccoli, chopped

★ 1 cup red or yellow bell pepper (1 large pepper), cut into 2" strips

2 cups yellow or green zucchini, cut into 2" strips

1 cup green onions, chopped

★ 2 cups fresh snow peas

2 cups canned cubed pineapple, drained

Option (to enhance the protein content):

Add 2 cups cubed firm low-fat tofu to stir-fry. For best results, freeze tofu, then thaw before cooking. Alternatively, use baked tofu or tofu packed in water, drained.

Directions

1. Dissolve cornstarch in water.
2. Combine all ingredients for sauce in a small pot. Cook over medium heat until sauce thickens. Remove from heat. Add tofu to sauce (optional).
3. Heat oil in wok or large cast-iron skillet.
4. Add vegetables and pineapple. Cook until vegetables are tender but crisp. Note: Dividing the amount of oil and vegetables into three parts and cooking each third separately can shorten the total cooking time and avoid overcooking of vegetables. Once each third is cooked, put cooked vegetables in a "holding" pan. Then combine all cooked vegetables with sauce.
5. Add sauce to cooked vegetables. Mix well.
6. Serve with brown rice or whole wheat couscous.

NUTRITION FACTS

Serving size 2 cups (stir-fry without rice)
Servings per recipe 4

Amount per serving
Calories 258   Calories from fat 59

Total Fat	6.5 grams
Saturated Fat	1 gram
Cholestrol	0 milligrams
Sodium	479 milligrams
Total Carbohydrate	48 grams
Dietary Fiber	8 grams
Sugars	18 grams
Protein	7 grams

Super nutrients: vitamins A, B, and C, folate, calcium, iron, magnesium, potassium

Recipe made with low-fat tofu: 308 calories, 8 grams total fat, and 16 grams protein

Sample Menu

Polynesian Stir-Fry
Served on a bed of steamed brown rice
Mango sorbet topped with fresh raspberries

Lentil Veggie Salad Combo

Protein and fiber-rich lentils offer a nutty taste and texture to a traditional garden salad.

Ingredients

★ ¾ cup dry brown or red lentils (time-saving tip: cook lentils in advance)

14-ounce can chicken or vegetable broth (can substitute reduced-sodium broth)

1 cup celery, finely diced (about 1 large stalk)

★ 1 cup carrots, finely diced

★ 1 cup tomato, finely diced

★ 1 cup yellow bell pepper, finely diced

1 cup red onion, finely diced (about half medium onion)

¼ cup reduced-fat red wine vinegar salad dressing (5 grams total fat/2 tablespoons serving indicated on label)

Salt or garlic salt to taste

¼ teaspoon pepper (or to taste)

Directions

1. Line colander with a paper towel. Top with lentils and rinse well.
2. Transfer washed lentils to saucepan. Add broth. Cook, covered, over medium heat for 30–40 minutes or until tender. Can add ¼–½ cup water, if necessary. Set aside.
3. In a large bowl, combine diced vegetables, salad dressing, salt, and pepper. Add cooked lentils. Mix well.
4. Serve lentil salad chilled over a bed of mixed, fresh greens.

<u>Sample</u> <u>Menu</u>

Lentil Veggie Salad Combo 🗒

Baked whole wheat pita triangles

Seasoned with garlic salt and cooking spray

Strawberry sundae

Nonfat vanilla yogurt topped with fresh

strawberries and nonfat chocolate syrup

NUTRITION FACTS

Serving size 1½ cups

Servings per recipe 4

Amount per serving

Calories 235   Calories from fat 63

Total Fat	7 grams
Saturated Fat	1 gram
Cholesterol	0 milligrams
Sodium*	747 milligrams
Total Carbohydrate	32 grams
Dietary Fiber	11 grams
Sugars	5 grams
Protein	13 grams

Super nutrients: vitamins A and C,

folate; iron, potassium

*Recipe prepared with reduced-sodium broth contains

510 milligrams sodium

Cajun Beans and Rice

A quick and easy meatless Southern fixin' showcasing okra, a commonly used vegetable in Cajun country.

Ingredients

1 large onion, chopped

2 tablespoons garlic, minced

Nonstick cooking spray

★ *1½ cups fresh okra, sliced crosswise, or 10-ounce package of frozen sliced okra, thawed*

★ *1 can (15 ounces) kidney or red beans, drained*

★ *1 can (15 ounces) black beans, drained*

2 cups cooked brown rice (1 cup dried brown rice + 2½ cups water)

★ *16-ounce can low-sodium tomato sauce*

½ teaspoon hot pepper sauce (or to taste)

½ teaspoon Cajun/Creole seasoning (or to taste)

Directions

1. Sauté onions and garlic in nonstick cooking spray.
2. In a large saucepan or skillet, combine all ingredients.
3. Cook over medium heat for 10 minutes until mixture is hot.

<u>Sample</u> <u>Menu</u>

Mixed field greens salad
with seasoned red wine vinegar
Cajun Beans and Rice ☑
Low-fat corn muffin
Caramel apple
Apple slices with nonfat caramel fruit dip

NUTRITION FACTS

Serving size 1½ cups
Servings per recipe 6

Amount per serving
Calories 325   Calories from fat 18

Total Fat	2 grams
Saturated Fat	0 grams
Cholesterol	0 milligrams
Sodium	702 milligrams
Total Carbohydrate	64 grams
Dietary Fiber	14 grams
Sugars	6 grams
Protein	17 grams

Super nutrients: vitamins B_6 and C,
folate; iron, magnesium, potassium

Super Meaty Main Events

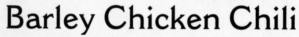

Barley Chicken Chili

Don't chicken out on this chili! Savor the refreshing flavor and texture that barley offers to this "white" chili.

Ingredients

1 large onion, finely chopped

2 tablespoons garlic, minced

★ ½ cup fresh or canned jalapeño peppers, finely chopped

1 tablespoon canola oil or olive oil

11-ounce can whole kernel corn, drained

½ cup dry pearl barley (do not use quick-cooking barley)

1 cup water

★ 2 cans (15.5 ounces each) diced tomatoes, with liquid

★ 15-ounce can black beans, drained (optional)

★ 15-ounce can tomato sauce

2 cans (15 ounces each) chicken broth (can substitute reduced-sodium chicken broth)

2 tablespoons chili powder (or to taste)

1 teaspoon ground cumin

3 cups (about 2 pounds) cooked, skinless chicken breast, cubed

Directions

1. Sauté onion, garlic, and jalapeño peppers with oil in a small frying pan.
2. In a large soup pot, combine sautéed vegetables with remaining ingredients except chicken. Bring to a boil.
3. Reduce heat to low. Cover pot and simmer for 40 minutes (or until barley is tender), stirring occasionally.
4. Add cubed chicken and cook an additional 10 minutes.
5. If chili is too thick, add water to reach desired consistency. Chili peaks in flavor 24–48 hours after preparation.

Sample Menu

Skinny Guacamole ▱
Served with raw vegetables and baked tortilla chips
Barley Chicken Chili ▱
Low-fat sandwich cookies

NUTRITION FACTS

Serving size 2 cups
Servings per recipe 9

Amount per serving
Calories 284   Calories from fat 45

Total Fat	5 grams
Saturated Fat	1 gram
Cholesterol	38 milligrams
Sodium*	1181 milligrams
Total Carbohydrate	38 grams
Dietary Fiber	7 grams
Sugars	5 grams
Protein	24 grams

Super nutrients: vitamins B$_6$ and C,
folate; magnesium, potassium

* 991 milligrams sodium using reduced-sodium chicken broth.

Turkey Loaf Florentine

Craving homemade "comfort" food? Try this Italian-style meatloaf stuffed with spinach.

Ingredients

Turkey Mixture:

Nonstick cooking spray

½ large yellow onion, chopped

1 pound 93% lean ground turkey (can substitute 93% lean ground beef), uncooked

¾ cup dry oats, uncooked

2 large egg whites, lightly beaten

2 teaspoons Italian blend of seasonings

¼ teaspoon garlic or onion salt (optional)

½ teaspoon black pepper

Spinach Stuffing:

2 cups white mushrooms, sliced

★ 10 ounces frozen chopped spinach, thawed and drained well

½ large yellow onion, chopped

¼ cup grated parmesan cheese

2 tablespoons minced garlic

Topping:

2 cups low-fat meatless spaghetti sauce (no more than 3 grams fat per ½ cup listed on label)

½ cup grated part-skim mozzarella cheese

Directions

1. Preheat oven to 375°. Spray an 11" × 7" glass loaf pan with nonfat cooking spray.

2. Sauté ½ onion in nonfat cooking spray.
3. Mix all ingredients for the turkey mixture in a large bowl. Set aside.
4. Sauté mushrooms using nonfat cooking spray.
5. In a separate bowl, combine sautéed mushrooms with all other ingredients for spinach filling. Mix well.
6. Spoon ⅔ of turkey mixture into the loaf pan, making a deep indentation down center.
7. Fill indentation with all of spinach stuffing.
8. Top with remaining turkey mixture, sealing edges to completely cover spinach filling with turkey.

NUTRITION FACTS

Serving size 1 slice
Servings per recipe 6

Amount per serving

Calories 281   Calories from fat 81

Total Fat	9 grams
Saturated Fat	3 grams
Cholesterol	58 milligrams
Sodium	544 milligrams
Total Carbohydrate	17 grams
Dietary Fiber	4 grams
Sugars	3 grams
Protein	26 grams

Super nutrients: vitamins A, B_6, and C, potassium; bonus from dairy: 200 milligrams calcium

9. Generously cover meatloaf with spaghetti sauce.
10. Cover with foil and bake 45–50 minutes or until cooked thoroughly.
11. During the last 5 minutes of cooking, remove cover and sprinkle loaf with mozzarella. Bake until cheese turns golden brown.
12. Let meatloaf stand 5 minutes before slicing.

Sample Menu

Turkey Loaf Florentine ☐
Steamed broccoli and cauliflower
Baked white potato with light sour cream
Jell-O fruit mold

Hawaiian Mango Salsa Salmon

Topping heart-healthy salmon with a taste of tropical paradise offers a zest of flavor and a splash of color.

Ingredients

Salsa:

⭐ *1 fresh mango, peeled and cubed*
⭐ *1 medium red bell pepper, cored and finely chopped*
2 medium green onions, finely chopped
1 tablespoon canola oil or olive oil
2 tablespoons lime juice
1 tablespoon vinegar
¼ cup fresh cilantro, finely chopped
  (optional)
Salt to taste

Salmon:

6 salmon fillets, 3 ounces each
  (Atlantic salmon is the richest
  source of omega-3 fats.)
Sesame seed oil (can substitute
  canola or olive oil)

Directions

1. Combine salsa ingredients in a small mixing bowl. Cover and chill for at least 1 hour.

NUTRITION FACTS

Salmon with Sesame Oil

Serving size 3-ounce fillet
Servings per recipe 6

Amount per serving	
Calories 164	Calories from fat 18

Total Fat	8 grams
Saturated Fat	1 gram
Cholesterol	60 milligrams
Sodium	48 milligrams
Total Carbohydrate	0 grams
Dietary Fiber	0 grams
Sugars	0 grams
Protein	22 grams

Bonus: 1.9 grams omega-3 fat from Atlantic salmon

2. Using a pastry brush or paper towel, lightly coat topside of each salmon fillet with ¼ teaspoon of sesame seed oil. Bake salmon for 15 minutes (or until fish "flakes" using the fork test) at 350°.

3. Top each cooked salmon fillet with ¼ cup chilled mango salsa just prior to serving.

NUTRITION FACTS	
Mango Salsa	
Serving size ¼ cup	
Servings per recipe 6	
Amount per serving	
Calories 51	Calories from fat 18
Total Fat	2 grams
Saturated Fat	0 grams
Cholesterol	0 milligrams
Sodium*	3 milligrams
Total Carbohydrate	8 grams
Dietary Fiber	1 gram
Sugars	5 grams
Protein	0 grams
Super nutrients: vitamins A and C	
*Indicates no salt added to recipe	

Sample Menu

Fresh spinach salad with light dressing
Hawaiian Mango Salsa Salmon
Steamed brown and wild rice
Lemon sorbet

Super Sides

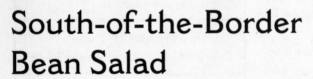

South-of-the-Border Bean Salad

This recipe is a spicier spin on a three-bean salad, chock-full of vegetables.

Ingredients

Bean Salad:
- ✭ 1 can (15 ounces) dark red kidney beans, drained
- ✭ 1 can (15 ounces) black beans, drained
- ✭ 1 can (15 ounces) garbanzo beans (chickpeas) drained
- ✭ 2 cups fresh tomatoes, diced
- 1 cup green or red onions, finely chopped
- 1 cup celery (3 large celery stalks), chopped
- ✭ 1 large red bell pepper, finely chopped
- 1 cup finely chopped fresh cilantro

Dressing:
- 1 tablespoon canola oil or olive oil
- 1/4 cup rice or red wine vinegar
- 3 tablespoons minced garlic
- 4 teaspoons chili powder
- 1/2 teaspoon ground cumin
- 1/2 teaspoon garlic salt (or to taste)

Directions

1. Combine all bean salad ingredients in a large bowl. Mix well.
2. Mix dressing ingredients thoroughly in a separate bowl.
3. Pour dressing on bean salad. Mix well.
4. Refrigerate several hours before serving. Marinate salad overnight for optimal flavor.

Sample Menu

South-of-the-Border Bean Salad ▢
Grilled lean hamburger
Served on a whole-grain bun
Baby carrots and celery sticks
Fudgsicle

NUTRITION FACTS

Serving size 1 cup
Servings per recipe 8

Amount per serving
Calories 237   Calories from fat 36

Total Fat	4 grams
Saturated Fat	0.5 gram
Cholesterol	0 milligrams
Sodium	660 milligrams
Total Carbohydrate	46 grams
Dietary Fiber	12 grams
Sugars	4 grams
Protein	15 grams

Super nutrients: vitamin C, folate;
iron

Asian Sesame Salad Greens

Bok choy, a member of the cabbage family, is a traditional vegetable used in Asian cooking. In this oriental tossed salad, toasted sesame seed dressing adds a nutty flavor.

Ingredients

Bok Choy Salad:

★ 1 head fresh bok choy (Napa cabbage), washed and chopped (white stalks and dark green leaves)

1 cup chopped green onion (about 2 large bunches)

★ 1 large red bell pepper, finely chopped

1 package Oriental flavor ramen noodles (uncooked), crumbled

Dressing:

2 tablespoons sesame seed oil or canola oil

¼ cup toasted sesame seeds (toast in toaster or conventional oven until golden brown)

¼ cup lemon juice

1 tablespoon granulated sugar

1 seasoning packet from the Oriental flavor ramen noodles listed above

¼ teaspoon onion salt (optional)

Directions

1. In a large salad bowl, combine all bok choy salad ingredients except ramen noodles.
2. In a separate bowl, combine ingredients for dressing. Mix well.
3. Pour dressing over salad. Using salad forks, thoroughly coat bok choy and other vegetables with dressing.
4. Sprinkle ramen noodles on salad. Serve immediately.
5. Salad may be refrigerated in a covered container up to 3 days. "Dressed" salad wilts with prolonged refrigeration.

Sample <u>M</u>enu

Moroccan Pumpkin Soup 📋
Grilled chicken breast
Asian Sesame Salad Greens 📋
Served with garlic-flavored melba toast
Frozen fruit juice bar

NUTRITION FACTS

Serving size 2 cups
Servings per recipe 8

Amount per serving
Calories 122   Calories from fat 68

Total Fat	7.5 grams
Saturated Fat	1.3 grams
Cholesterol	0 milligrams
Sodium	259 milligrams
Total Carbohydrate	12 grams
Dietary Fiber	2.5 grams
Sugars	3 grams
Protein	4 grams
Super nutrients: vitamins A and C, folate	

Sunshine Bell Pepper Salad

Enjoy the kaleidoscope of colors and flavors in this multivegetable salad.

Ingredients

★ *1 cup garbanzo beans (chickpeas), drained*

★ *½ cup fresh parsley, finely chopped*

1 cup (1 small) red onion, finely chopped

★ *1 large red bell pepper, cored and finely chopped*

★ *1 large yellow or orange bell pepper, cored and finely chopped*

½ cup cucumber with skin, chopped

2 tablespoons balsamic vinegar

3 tablespoons light red wine vinegar dressing (no more than 5 grams total fat per 2-tablespoon serving indicated on label)

¼ teaspoon each garlic salt and black pepper (or to taste)

Directions

1. Combine all ingredients in a large bowl. Mix well.
2. Cover and refrigerate several hours before serving.
3. Salad keeps up to 3 days in the refrigerator.

Sample Menu

Low-fat tuna salad sandwich
Served on whole wheat bread
Sunshine Bell Pepper Salad 📖
Fresh fruit salad

NUTRITION FACTS	
Serving size 1 cup	
Servings per recipe 4	
Amount per serving	
Calories 155	Calories from fat 50
Total Fat	5.5 grams
Saturated Fat	1 gram
Cholesterol	0 milligrams
Sodium	317 milligrams
Total Carbohydrate	23 grams
Dietary Fiber	6 grams
Sugars	5.5 grams
Protein	6 grams
Super nutrients: vitamins A and C, folate	

Quinoa Fruitopia

Take a virtual culinary expedition to the Andes Mountains with a delicate grain grown exclusively in South America. Quinoa (keen-wha) was considered sacred by the ancient Incas.

Ingredients

Quinoa:

1 cup dried quinoa (found in the rice or specialty foods section of large supermarkets)

2 cups water

¼ teaspoon salt

5 medium green onions (white part only), finely chopped

1 cup (2–3 large stalks) celery, diced

Nonstick cooking spray

★ ½ cup dried apricot halves or dried papaya, or a combination, finely chopped

½ cup dried cranberries or raisins

★ 1 cup fresh oranges, peeled and white rind removed, diced (can substitute chopped mandarin oranges)

★ 1 large yellow bell pepper, cored and finely chopped (can substitute green pepper)

Dressing:

2 tablespoons lemon or lime juice

1 teaspoon white sugar

¼ cup fresh cilantro, finely chopped (optional)

¼ teaspoon paprika

¼ teaspoon mild curry powder

¼ teaspoon ground cumin

¼ teaspoon ground ginger

¼ teaspoon ground cinnamon

2 teaspoons olive oil or canola oil

⅛ teaspoon salt (or to taste)

Directions

1. Line a colander with a paper towel. Top with quinoa and rinse well.

2. In a medium-size saucepan, bring water and salt to a boil. Add quinoa. Lower the heat and cook covered for 15 minutes or until all the water is absorbed (quinoa is thoroughly cooked when it's translucent and the germ is visible).

3. Sauté onions and celery in a small frying pan sprayed with nonstick cooking spray.

4. In a large mixing bowl, combine cooked quinoa with fruit and sautéed vegetables.

5. In a small bowl, combine all the dressing ingredients. Mix well.

6. Add dressing to quinoa-vegetable mixture. Mix well.

7. Cover and refrigerate several hours before serving. Salad peaks in flavor 24 hours after preparation.

NUTRITION FACTS

Serving size 1 cup
Servings per recipe 5

Amount per serving
Calories 237   Calories from fat 36

Total Fat	4 grams
Saturated Fat	0.5 grams
Cholesterol	0 milligrams
Sodium	211 milligrams
Total Carbohydrate	49 grams
Dietary Fiber	5 grams
Sugars	11 grams
Protein	6 grams

Super nutrients: vitamin C; iron, magnesium, potassium

Sample Menu

Mixed field greens
with seasoned rice wine vinegar
Grilled turkey burger
Served on a whole-grain bun
Quinoa Fruitopia
Popsicle

California Jicama Salad

Jicama, a Mexican raw "potato," adds crunch to this salad blend, which contains a colorful array of Mother Nature's finest plant foods.

Ingredients

Salad:

★ *2 cups (about 1 medium) raw jicama, peeled, cut in ½" cubes*

★ *2 cups cantaloupe, cubed*

1½ cups (1 medium) cucumber with skin, cut lengthwise, seeded and cubed

1 cup finely chopped fresh cilantro

¾ cup dried cranberries (craisins)

★ *⅓ cup roasted almonds, slivered (optional)*

Dressing:

2 tablespoons lime juice

★ *2 tablespoons orange juice concentrate, undiluted*

2 tablespoons granulated sugar

½ teaspoon salt

1 tablespoon chili powder

Directions

1. Combine all salad ingredients except almonds in a medium-size salad bowl.
2. In a small mixing bowl, mix dressing ingredients well.
3. Pour dressing on salad. Mix well.
4. Toast almonds in toaster oven until golden brown. Sprinkle on top before serving.
5. Salad will remain fresh for 2 days refrigerated.

<u>Sample</u> <u>Menu</u>

Baked Swiss Chard Frittata 🗇
California Jicama Salad 🗇
Crusty whole wheat roll
Fat-free raspberry Newtons

NUTRITION FACTS

Serving size 1 cup
Servings per recipe 7

Amount per serving
Calories 134   Calories from fat 27

Total Fat	3 grams
Saturated Fat	0 grams
Cholesterol	0 milligrams
Sodium	180 milligrams
Total Carbohydrate	28 grams
Dietary Fiber	4 grams
Sugars	17 grams
Protein	2 grams
Super nutrients: vitamins A and C	

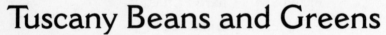

Tuscany Beans and Greens

The sweetness from the tomatoes and shallots takes the "bite" out of cooked greens in this less common Italian dish.

Ingredients

1 cup diced shallots (can substitute white onion)

2 tablespoons minced garlic

1 tablespoon olive oil or canola oil

1 tablespoon granulated sugar

★ *1 can (15 ounces) diced tomatoes, unseasoned, drained*

★ *1 can (15.5 ounces) cannellini (white Italian) beans, drained*

★ *4 cups cooked fresh greens, or frozen greens, chopped, defrosted (for best results, use a blend of turnip, mustard, and collard greens)*

¼ teaspoon salt (or to taste)

¼ teaspoon white pepper

¼ cup parmesan cheese

Directions

1. Sauté shallots and garlic with olive oil.
2. In a medium-size pot, combine sautéed shallots and garlic with remaining ingredients except parmesan cheese.
3. Cook until mixture comes to a light boil.
4. Remove from heat and immediately stir in parmesan cheese.

<u>Sample</u> <u>Menu</u>

Tossed green salad with light dressing
Baked halibut
Seasoned with lemon and fresh herbs
Tuscany Beans and Greens ☙
Crusty whole-grain roll
Lemon sorbet
Topped with fresh raspberries

NUTRITION FACTS

Serving size 1 cup
Servings per recipe 6

Amount per serving
Calories 203   Calories from fat 36

Total Fat	4 grams
Saturated Fat	1 gram
Cholesterol	3 milligrams
Sodium	552 milligrams
Total Carbohydrate	32 grams
Dietary Fiber	9 grams
Sugars	4 grams
Protein	12 grams

Super nutrients: vitamins A and C,
folate; potassium; bonus from vegetables
and cheese: 278 milligrams calcium

Cranbroccoli Salad

Sunflower seeds significantly enhance the nutritional value of this creamy broccoli salad.

Ingredients

Salad:

★ *5 cups raw broccoli flowerets, chopped in small pieces*
½ cup (about 1 small) red onion, finely chopped
★ *¼ cup salted dry-roasted sunflower seeds*
¾ cup dried cranberries (craisins)

Dressing:

2 tablespoons granulated sugar
1 cup low-fat mayonnaise
2 tablespoons red wine vinegar
1 teaspoon liquid smoke (optional)
¼ teaspoon salt (or to taste)
⅛ teaspoon pepper

Directions

1. Combine salad ingredients in a medium-size salad bowl. Mix well.
2. In a small bowl, mix dressing ingredients well.
3. Pour dressing into salad. Mix until vegetables are lightly covered with dressing.
4. Cover and chill for at least an hour before serving.

Sample Menu

Turkey cheese sandwich
Turkey breast, light Swiss cheese,
and mustard on pumpernickel bread
Cranbroccoli Salad 📋
Gingersnaps

NUTRITION FACTS

Serving size 1 cup
Servings per recipe 7

Amount per serving
Calories 163   Calories from fat 45

Total Fat	5 grams
Saturated Fat	1 gram
Cholesterol	0 milligrams
Sodium	454 milligrams
Total Carbohydrate	30 grams
Dietary Fiber	3 grams
Sugars	14 grams
Protein	3 grams
Super nutrients: vitamins C and E	

Kale 'n' Mushrooms

Bring kale, a member of the cruciferous vegetable family, out of its "hiding" as a garnish. This dark green leafy vegetable is nutrition dynamite!

Ingredients

2 cups sliced raw mushrooms

1 teaspoon canola oil or olive oil

★ *8 cups fresh green or purple (Russian) kale, washed*

2 tablespoons balsamic vinegar

1 teaspoon sesame oil (can substitute canola or olive oil)

1 teaspoon granulated sugar

¼ teaspoon garlic salt

Directions

1. Sauté mushrooms with oil in a medium-size skillet. Set aside.
2. Tear leaves from midrib of kale. Steam kale for about 5 minutes or until leaves turn a dark color and are tender.
3. In a small bowl, mix vinegar, oil, sugar, and salt.
4. Combine mushrooms, kale, and dressing in a skillet and mix well. Cook on low heat for 1 minute or until hot. Note: Overcooked kale turns a lighter color and tastes bitter.

<u>Sample</u> <u>Menu</u>

Tossed green salad
with seasoned red wine vinegar
Eggplant et Cetera Parmesan ▱
Served on a bed of whole wheat pasta
Kale 'n' Mushrooms ▱
Low-fat lemon cookies

NUTRITION FACTS

Serving size 1 cup
Servings per recipe 3

Amount per serving
Calories 107   Calories from fat 36

Total Fat	4 grams
Saturated Fat	0.5 gram
Cholesterol	0 milligrams
Sodium	111 milligrams
Total Carbohydrate	15 grams
Dietary Fiber	5 grams
Sugars	3 grams
Protein	7 grams

Super nutrients: vitamins A and C,
calcium, potassium

Summer Spinach Salad

Popeye would savor this fruited spinach salad.

Ingredients

Salad:

★ *1 package (10 ounces) fresh baby spinach, washed, torn into bite-size pieces*

★ *½ pint fresh raspberries or strawberries, sliced*

★ *4 medium kiwi, peeled, sliced crosswise*

1½ cups red or Concord seedless grapes, cut in halves

★ *1 large orange, peeled and sectioned, cut into bite-size pieces*

★ *½ cup unsalted slivered almonds or walnuts*

Raspberry Yogurt Dressing:

1 cup nonfat plain yogurt

★ *½ cup fresh or frozen raspberries*

¼ cup balsamic vinegar

2 tablespoons honey (or to taste)

Directions

1. Line a large salad bowl with washed and torn spinach leaves.
2. Equally spread the fruits on top of spinach.
3. Toast almonds in toaster oven or conventional oven until golden brown (1–5 minutes). (If used as a substitution, walnuts do not need to be toasted.)

NUTRITION FACTS	
Spinach Salad	
Serving size 2 cups	
Servings per recipe 7	
Amount per serving	
Calories 146	Calories from fat 18
Total Fat	5 grams
Saturated Fat	0.5 gram
Cholesterol	0 milligrams
Sodium	33 milligrams
Total Carbohydrate	25 grams
Dietary Fiber	5 grams
Sugars	11 grams
Protein	4 grams
Super nutrients: vitamins A and C, folate	

4. Sprinkle nuts on top of salad.
5. Refrigerate salad until ready to serve.
6. Mix all dressing ingredients in a blender until smooth.
7. Individually pour 2 tablespoons dressing on each portion of salad immediately prior to serving.

NUTRITION FACTS
Raspberry Yogurt Dressing
Serving size 2 tablespoons
Servings per recipe 8

Amount per serving
Calories 38   Calories from fat 18

Total Fat	0 grams
Saturated Fat	0 grams
Cholesterol	0.5 milligrams
Sodium	24 milligrams
Total Carbohydrate	8 grams
Dietary Fiber	0.5 grams
Sugars	3 grams
Protein	2 grams

Sample Menu

Summer Spinach Salad
Baked orange roughy
Seasoned with fresh herbs
Brown rice pilaf
Carrot Cake DeLITE

Super Sweets

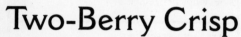

Two-Berry Crisp

A "berry" healthy alternative to blueberry pie, sprinkled with ground flaxseed, a rich plant source of heart-smart omega-3 fats.

Ingredients

Berry Mixture:
Nonstick cooking spray
★ *2 cups fresh or frozen blackberries, thawed*
2 cups fresh or frozen blueberries, thawed
2 tablespoons lemon juice

Oat Topping:
⅔ cup dry oats
⅓ cup all-purpose flour
★ *2 tablespoons ground flaxseed (use coffee grinder to grind whole flaxseeds)*
½ cup packed dark brown sugar
1 teaspoon cinnamon
3 tablespoons light tub margarine (no more than 5 grams fat/tablespoon per label)

Directions

1. Spray a 7" × 11" brownie pan with nonstick cooking spray.
2. Evenly spread berries in pan. Sprinkle with lemon juice.
3. In a small mixing bowl, combine oat topping ingredients with a fork until mixture resembles small peas.
4. Spread oat topping to cover the berries.
5. Bake uncovered at 400° for 15–20 minutes or until berries are bubbly. Serve hot. Serving suggestion: Top with ¼ cup nonfat vanilla yogurt (an additional 40 calories).

<u>Sample</u> <u>Menu</u>

Garden salad with light dressing
Cruciferous Veggie Casserole 🗂
Pumpernickel roll
Two-Berry Crisp 🗂

NUTRITION FACTS

Serving size ½ cup
Servings per recipe 8

Amount per serving
Calories 175   Calories from fat 27

Total Fat	3 grams
Saturated Fat	0.5 gram
Cholesterol	0 milligrams
Sodium	46 milligrams
Total Carbohydrate	35 grams
Dietary Fiber	5 grams
Sugars	17 grams
Protein	3 grams

Super nutrients: vitamin C; bonus:
0.5 gram omega-3 fats from flaxseed

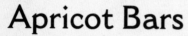

Apricot Bars

This chewy fruit cookie satisfies your sweet tooth for fewer calories than an apricot sweet roll.

Ingredients

Apricot Topping:

★ *2½ cups dried apricot halves, finely chopped*
★ *⅓ cup orange juice concentrate*
⅓ cup water
¼ cup honey

Crust:

1 cup whole wheat flour
½ cup all-purpose white flour
½ cup light tub margarine (no more than 5 grams fat/tablespoon per label)
¾ cup firmly packed brown sugar
1 teaspoon cinnamon
Nonstick cooking spray

Directions

1. Cook apricot topping ingredients in a saucepan over medium heat until mixture boils.
2. Reduce heat to low and cook for an additional 20–25 minutes or until mixture has thickened (resembling chunky apricot preserves).
3. While apricot mixture is cooking, combine crust ingredients in a small mixing bowl. Using a fork, coat the flour mixture with the light tub margarine until the mixture resembles the consistency of small peas. Note: Overhandling flour mixture may result in a tough crust.

4. Pat the flour crust mixture evenly in a 7" × 11" brownie pan 'greased' with nonstick cooking spray.

5. Pour thickened apricot mixture on top of crust and bake at 350° for 20 minutes.

6. Cool completely. Cut into 12 bars.

NUTRITION FACTS

Serving size 1 bar
Servings per recipe 12

Amount per serving
Calories 215   Calories from fat 36

Total Fat	4 grams
Saturated Fat	0.5 grams
Cholesterol	0 milligrams
Sodium	72 milligrams
Total Carbohydrate	45 grams
Dietary Fiber	3 grams
Sugars	22 grams
Protein	3 grams

Super nutrients: vitamin A, potassium

Sample Menu

Tossed green salad
with seasoned rice wine vinegar
Spinach Lasagna Supreme 🗇
Garlic bread made with light tub margarine
Apricot Bars 🗇

Carrot Cake DeLITE

This skinnier version of a traditional dessert favorite is flavored with orange zest and spices (calories reduced by half; total fat decreased by two-thirds).

Ingredients

Cake:

Nonstick cooking spray

4 large egg whites

1 whole large egg (Note: can use commercial egg substitute but yields a denser cake texture)

1 cup brown sugar

1/2 cup granulated sugar

1/2 cup canola oil

1 cup applesauce

1 tablespoon freshly grated orange peel (zest or rind from one medium orange)

1 teaspoon cinnamon

1/2 teaspoon nutmeg

★ 3 cups grated carrots

3 cups all-purpose white flour

1 teaspoon baking powder

1 teaspoon baking soda

Frosting:

6 ounces light cream cheese

3 cups powdered sugar (per desired consistency)

1 teaspoon vanilla extract

Directions

1. Preheat oven to 325°. Grease bundt pan with nonstick cooking spray.
2. Beat eggs whites and egg with a wire whisk. Add sugars, oil, applesauce. Mix well.

3. Add orange peel and spices. Mix well.
4. Mix in grated carrots.
5. In a separate bowl, combine flour, baking powder, and baking soda. Mix well.
6. Carefully add flour to egg mixture by mixing with a large spoon until all the flour is moistened. Note: Overmixing the batter will cause the cake to be tough.
7. Pour batter into pan and bake about 45 minutes or until toothpick in center comes out clean.
8. Immediately, run a butter knife around the edges of the pan for easier removal. Allow cake to cool in pan for ONLY 10 minutes. Invert cake onto serving platter.
9. Using an electric mixer, beat cream cheese until fluffy. Gradually add powdered sugar and vanilla until mixture resembles desired frosting consistency.
10. Frost cake and cut into 16 slices.

NUTRITION FACTS

Serving size 1 slice
Servings per recipe 16

Amount per serving

Calories 335   Calories from fat 81

Total Fat	9 grams
Saturated Fat	2 grams
Cholesterol	19 milligrams
Sodium	190 milligrams
Total Carbohydrate	65 grams
Dietary Fiber	1 gram
Sugars	43 grams
Protein	5 grams
Super nutrient: vitamin A	

Sample Menu

Summer Spinach Salad
Baked orange roughy
Seasoned with fresh herbs
Brown rice pilaf
Carrot Cake DeLITE

Super Food Nutrients
(essential for health but lacking in the typical American diet)

Vitamins	Minerals	Fiber	Phytochemicals
■ Vitamins A, C, and E are antioxidants that may play a role in warding off heart disease and certain cancers. ■ High intake of vitamin B6 and folate is associated with reduced risk of heart disease.	■ Calcium is important for bone health and blood pressure control. ■ Magnesium and potassium can help lower blood pressure. ■ Adequate intakes of iron can reduce the risk of iron-deficiency anemia, especially among younger women and children.	■ Higher-fiber diets promote successful weight loss and long-term maintenance of a healthy body weight. ■ A high-fiber diet is associated with a reduced risk of heart disease, cancer, and diabetes.	■ Hundreds of phytochemicals work synergistically to boost immunity, fight disease, and improve overall health. ■ Phytochemicals exhibit healthful effects on the body, such as reducing inflammation, lowering blood cholesterol, and fighting viruses or bacteria.

The phytochemicals are another health bonus of consuming a calorie-controlled diet rich in super foods. Although phytochemicals (phyto=plant; chemicals=natural substances) are technically not nutrients, these health-promoting substances may ward off disease (hence, they are descriptively known as "disease-fighting substances"). The table below describes the most common kinds of phytochemicals classified by color with their corresponding potential health benefits. You should consume a wide variety of phytochemicals by eating a spectrum of colorful plant foods. Since this is an emerging area of nutrition research, the information in this table is just the tip of the iceberg.

Super Food Phytochemicals

Fruits	Plant Pigments	Phytochemicals	Potential Health Benefits
Apricot, mango, cantaloupe	Orange	Beta-carotene	Antioxidant, boosts immunity, improves lung function, may slow the aging process, reduces cancer risk
Berries	Red, blue, purple	Ellagic acid, anthocyanins	Reduce cancer risk, lower blood cholesterol, reduce risk of blood clotting
Grapes, red	Red, purple	Resveratrol, quercetins	Reduce risk of heart disease, cancer, and blood clotting; anti-inflammatory
Kiwi	Green	Beta-carotene, lutein, ellagic acid, anthocyanins	Improve vision, lung function, and immunity; lower blood cholesterol; reduce risk of blood clotting and macular degeneration
Orange and other citrus	Orange, yellow	Flavonoids, limonene	Reduce risk of heart disease and certain cancers; improve lung function
Raisins, currants	Dark brown	Phenolic compounds	Antioxidants, may slow the aging process
Vegetables			
Asparagus, okra, green or snow peas, green or jalapeño pepper	Green	Beta-carotene, lutein (present in small amounts)	Antioxidants, boost immunity, improve lung function, improve vision, reduce cancer risk
Bok choy, broccoli, Brussels sprouts, cauliflower, kale, Swiss chard, greens (collard, mustard, turnip)	Dark green	Beta-carotene, lutein, sulphoraaphane, indoles	Antioxidants, boost immunity, reduce cancer risk, improve vision
Carrot	Orange	Beta-carotene	Antioxidant, boosts immunity, improves lung function, may slow the aging process, reduces cancer risk

Super Food Phytochemicals (cont.)

Vegetables	Plant Pigments	Phytochemicals	Potential Health Benefits
Corn	Yellow	Zeaxanthin	Improves vision and reduces risk of macular degeneration
Eggplant (skin)	Purple	Anthocyanins	May slow the aging process and reduce risk of urinary tract infections
Garlic, onions, leeks, scallions	White	Quercetins, allium compounds	Reduce risk of heart disease (lower blood cholesterol) and certain cancers
Parsley, cilantro	Green	Beta-carotene	Antioxidants, boost immunity, improve lung function, may slow the aging process, reduce cancer risk
Peppers, red	Red	Beta-carotene, lycopene	Antioxidant, boost immunity, improve lung function, may slow the aging process, reduce risk of heart disease and certain cancers
Spinach	Dark green	Beta-carotene, lutein, zeaxanthin	Antioxidant, boosts immunity, improves lung function, may slow the aging process, reduces risk of heart disease and certain cancers; may improve vision and reduce risk of macular degeneration
Sweet potato, butternut squash	Orange	Beta-carotene	Antioxidants, boost immunity, improve lung function, may slow the aging process, reduce cancer risk
Tomatoes, tomato sauce	Red	Lycopene	Reduce risk of heart disease and certain cancers

Nuts, Seeds, Oils	Plant Pigments	Phytochemicals	Potential Health Benefits
Nuts, seeds, oils	Yellow-brown	Ellagic acid, lignans, phytosterols	Antioxidants, lower blood cholesterol, reduce risk of heart disease and certain cancers
Grains, Dried Beans, Legumes			
Barley, oats, quinoa, whole wheat, brown rice	White-brown	Flavonoids, lignans	Antioxidants, lower blood cholesterol, reduce risk of heart disease and certain cancers
Lentils; dried garbanzo, black, kidney, red beans	Red, brown, black	Lignans, saponins	Help regulate blood sugar and blood cholesterol levels
Soybeans (in the form of tofu, TVP, or whole soybeans)	Light brown	Isoflavones (genestein and daidzein), lignans	May reduce risk of heart disease and certain hormone-dependent cancers

Chapter 8

Getting the Help
You Need

W hen it comes to weight loss, advertisements for effortless solutions can easily overshadow the many credible resources that are available. But they are there. You just may need a little help finding them.

Just as for other medical conditions, individual professional help by a licensed registered dietitian, psychologist, or physician is available for those who need or desire it. Formal weight loss programs or self-help groups can provide a different kind of structure, support, and accountability that some people need to ensure their success. The key is to know when to ask for help, what kind of help is available, which help is best for you, and how to find help that's reputable.

Nutritional Help

All dieters would probably benefit from a consultation with a registered dietitian (RD). Dietitians are uniquely qualified to perform a personalized nutritional assessment and counsel you on a diet that is individualized to your particular needs—an invaluable resource to my program and patients. Consider making an appointment to see a registered dietitian for the following:

- You need more help with meal planning, shopping, and preparation.
- You have special needs that require a tailored nutritional plan, such as diabetes, high blood cholesterol, high blood pressure, food allergies, or a gastrointestinal disease.

- You are interested in learning more about nutrition—including calories, nutrient composition, vitamins, minerals, phytochemicals, and the role of dietary supplements.
- You have been suffering from an eating disorder.

How to Find a Registered Dietitian

To contact an RD in your area, call the Consumer Nutrition Hotline of the American Dietetic Association at 1-800-366-1655 for a referral, or visit the ADA Web site at at www.eatright.org. Call your local hospital or ask your health care provider for a referral to an RD. Before your first visit, keep a food diary for two weekdays and the weekend. This way the nutritionist can help you analyze your eating habits and spot any nutritional deficiencies. After your first visit, you can decide whether more than just one session would be beneficial.

Psychological Help

Though many common, emotion-related eating issues can be dealt with by the coping strategies in Chapter 5, the following three conditions in particular may point to a need for psychological counseling:

- eating disorders, specifically binge eating disorder (BED) and bulimia nervosa
- emotional problems related to body image disturbance and low self-esteem
- mood disturbances such as depression

As you begin to pay attention to your eating, exercise, and coping patterns, you may uncover other psychological and behavioral problems, such as anxiety, obsessive-compulsive disorder (OCD), drug or alcohol abuse, and anorexia nervosa. Help is available for all these conditions and should be sought.

Binge Eating Disorder

Though food binges now and then are not uncommon and not a disorder (particularly when on vacation or at a party), bingeing behavior is a problem and diagnosable as binge eating disorder when it is characterized by the following three key features:

- *recurrent* episodes of binge eating (occurs, on average, at least 2 days a week for 6 months)
- feelings associated with a lack of control over eating (often feeling disgusted with yourself, depressed, or very guilty after overeating)
- being distressed about the behavior such that it interferes with your relationships with other people, with work, and with your ability to feel good about yourself

Using a combination of psychotherapy and medications, bingeing behavior can be brought under control, once it is recognized and treated.

Bulimia Nervosa

The symptoms that characterize bulimia nervosa overlap with BED. Both disorders are distinguished by recurrent episodes of binge eating associated with a lack of control. However, individuals with bulimia nervosa also engage in recurrent, inappropriate compensatory behavior in order to prevent weight gain, such as self-induced vomiting, misuse of laxatives or water pills, fasting, or excessive exercise. Bulimia means "eating like an ox." Individuals often plan the bulimic episodes—often triggered by anxiety, tension, or boredom—to correspond with specific binge foods, typically fatty, sweet, high-energy foods that they deny themselves at other times. The compensatory behavior, such as vomiting, is the result of feeling disgusted with themselves for having overeaten. This is a serious problem that can be helped with professional care.

Emotional Problems Related to Body Image Disturbance and Low Self-Esteem

It is very common for overweight people to be conscious about their body and shape. In fact, I consider that to be the norm. Individuals with a true body image disturbance, however, are overly dissatisfied with their appearance to the point that they are self-conscious in public or don't go out at all, are self-conscious in private especially in the bedroom, and have associated feelings of depression and low self-esteem. The mirror is avoided at all costs. Many of my patients with body image disturbance express the most hurtful, self-deprecating, and loathsome comments about themselves— remarks that underlie the pain and shame they feel about their body and shape. A central component of a condition called body dysmorphic disorder (BDD) is body image disturbance that involves an excessive preoccupation with a minor physical flaw or even an imagined defect in appearance. Here, excessive checking of the perceived flaw in the mirror is common. If you relate to having feelings of body image disturbance and low self-esteem that seriously impair your social functioning, professional help from a licensed psychologist or psychiatrist familiar with these issues is available.

Disturbances in Mood

When I meet patients for the first time, it is common for them to express a wide range of emotions when it comes to talking about their weight loss journey, including frustration, disappointment, anxiety, and sadness. These feelings typically come and go and are handled fairly well. However, if these emotional states linger, become overwhelming, and cloud all of your thoughts, you may be clinically depressed.

Clinical depression is characterized by long periods of sadness, markedly diminished interest or pleasure in all or almost all activities, fatigue or loss of energy, feelings of worthlessness or excessive guilt, and diminished ability to think or concentrate. These symptoms cause significant distress or impairment in social, occupational, or other important areas of your life. Although many people hope that losing weight will cure their depression, this rarely occurs. In this situation, treatment for the underlying depression must come first. If you think you have symptoms of clinical depression, my recommendation is to talk with your doctor about being referred to a psychologist or psychiatrist, or being treated with an antidepressant medication.

How to Find Psychological Help

To find a licensed psychologist or psychiatrist in your area, I recommend that you ask your primary health care provider for a referral. You can also try calling local hospitals. Before making an appointment, feel free to interview the psychologist or psychiatrist on the phone regarding his or her experience in your area of concern. You can also call the American Psychological Association at 1-800-964-2000 for referral to a mental health professional.

Medical Help

Overall, I recommend that all individuals who are overweight or obese see a physician at some point for a complete history and physical examination, particularly before beginning an exercise program. This is important since many ailments associated with obesity may be silent, most notably diabetes, high blood pressure (hypertension), and elevated blood fats. Other medical problems are symptomatic, such as shortness of breath, sleeping disturbances, heartburn, and pain in the weight-bearing joints. If these or other medical problems are present, you will need a doctor to treat and monitor them during your course of weight loss. Rarely, weight gain and obesity are caused by other medical or glandular diseases that may need to be explored as well. Another reason to see a doctor is if you have experienced unexpected weight gain after taking a medication such as those commonly prescribed for diabetes or mood disorders. Oftentimes, these medications can be substituted with others that are weight neutral. Lastly, you will need to see a doctor if you are interested in exploring the use of antiobesity medication or surgery as an aid for weight loss.

How to Find a Medical Physician

Start with your own doctor by asking him or her a few key questions:

- What is your attitude toward and experience with helping patients to lose weight?
- What would you recommend I do to lose weight?
- How would you work with me?
- Are you interested in and willing to partner with me for a weight loss plan?

Talking with your doctor will help you to evaluate your comfort level and confidence in his or her ability to help you. If, however, you prefer to find a doctor who specializes in obesity, you need to do your homework and be selective. There are very few formal training programs for the specialty of obesity. Some physicians (like myself) have undergone formal training in nutrition and are board certified. Some physicians are members of the American Society of Bariatric Physicians, which is a group of licensed physicians who offer specialized programs in the medical treatment of obesity or bariatrics (see Appendix C). The reality, however, is that most physicians who practice obesity care have acquired an interest in the field and established weight management programs on their own. Again, I encourage you to interview them on the phone before making your appointment.

Formal Programs

If you need more structure and accountability to support your behavior change, a formal weight loss program that incorporates nutritional information may also be helpful. You can check either local hospitals or outpatient physician practices that specialize in weight control or commercial weight management programs, many of which provide weekly weigh-ins, group meetings, personal encouragement, and reinforcement (such as Weight Watchers). Prior to signing up with any program, ask a few key questions as suggested by the Federal Trade Commission:

- What are the staff qualifications and central components of the program (program content and goals, frequency of visits, group versus individual care, staff's training, experience, certification, and education)?
- Are there any risks associated with the product or program (drugs, dietary supplements, diet, expected rate of weight loss, and monitoring)?
- What are the program costs?

Self-Help Groups

If you're interested in finding a support group, I can recommend these Web sites: Overeaters Anonymous at www.overeatersanonymous.org and TOPS (Take Off Pounds Sensibly) at www.tops.org. OA is a recovery program for overeating. TOPS is a support group that discusses the challenges and successes of losing weight. Member volunteers run both groups. While many people find these programs helpful in providing social support and accountability, others are dissatisfied with the lack of specific diet and exercise recommendations.

In addition, there's always a role for continual self-learning. Check out the list of books, magazines, and Web sites in Appendix C. The more information you have, the more successful you will be. Although this book is primarily intended for self-help purposes, it can be an excellent supplement to professional help as well. I encourage you to share this book, your patterns, and your strategies with any professionals who help you on your weight loss journey.

■　■　■　■　■

Appendix A
Your Body Mass Index (BMI)

■   ■   ■   ■   ■

Know Your BMI

Knowing your BMI and waist circumference is as important as knowing your blood pressure reading or cholesterol level. Since the risk of developing medical problems escalates with increasing body weight, it is useful to categorize your weight and associated risk level. Patients often ask me what they should weigh for improved or optimal health. You may be familiar with older terms such as "ideal body weight" or "desirable body weight." This terminology is no longer used. A more practical measurement of overweight and obesity is the body mass index, or BMI. BMI is calculated using a mathematical formula based on your height and weight. This term predicts the development of health problems related to excess weight. The higher your BMI, the greater your risk for developing diabetes, high blood pressure, some forms of cancer, osteoarthritis, sleep disturbances, stroke, and heart disease, among others. Although BMI compares well to the percentage of body fat, it is not a direct measurement of body fat. To determine your BMI, use the table on pages 267–268. Look down the left column to find your height (in inches) and then look across that row and find the weight that's nearest your own. Now look to the top of the column to find the number that is your BMI. For example, if you are 5'4" (64" tall) and weigh 164 pounds, your BMI is 28.

A BMI from 18.5 through 24.9 is desirable and healthy. The goal here is to prevent any further weight gain. A BMI from 25 through 29.9 is considered overweight and carries a slightly increased risk of weight-related health problems. A BMI of 30 or more is medically designated as obesity and carries a high risk for health-related problems. Morbid or severe obesity is regarded as a BMI of 40 or greater.

Please note that this tool is not exact. If you are highly active and muscular, your BMI may be higher than recommended. In this case, you should have a body fat analysis done by either skin fold anthropometry or bioimpedence analyses at a health club or a health care provider's office.

Independent of BMI, a large waist circumference increases the risk for developing health-related problems. The larger your waist, the greater the risk. If your BMI is between 25 and 34.9, measure your waist circumference horizontally at the level of your upper hip bone (pelvis). This can be done using a paper or cloth measuring tape, the one that tailors use. If your waist is greater than 40 inches (for men) or greater than 35 inches (for women), you have an even higher risk for diabetes, high blood pressure, elevated blood fats, and heart disease compared to people with lower waist circumferences. As you work through this program and lose weight, look forward to seeing an improvement in these health parameters.

BMI

BMI	19	20	21	22	23	24	25	26	27	28	29	30	31	32	33	34	35
Height (inches)								Body Weight (pounds)									
58	91	96	100	105	110	115	119	124	129	134	138	143	148	153	158	162	167
59	94	99	104	109	114	119	124	128	133	138	143	148	153	158	163	168	173
60	97	102	107	112	118	123	128	133	138	143	148	153	158	163	168	174	179
61	100	106	111	116	122	127	132	137	143	148	153	158	164	169	174	180	185
62	104	109	115	120	126	131	136	142	147	153	158	164	169	175	180	186	191
63	107	113	118	124	130	135	141	146	152	158	163	169	175	180	186	191	197
64	110	116	122	128	134	140	145	151	157	163	169	174	180	186	192	197	204
65	114	120	126	132	138	144	150	156	162	168	174	180	186	192	198	204	210
66	118	124	130	136	142	148	155	161	167	173	179	186	192	198	204	210	216
67	121	127	134	140	146	153	159	166	172	178	185	191	198	204	211	217	223
68	125	131	138	144	151	158	164	171	177	184	190	197	203	210	216	223	230
69	128	135	142	149	155	162	169	176	182	189	196	203	209	216	223	230	236
70	132	139	146	153	160	167	174	181	188	195	202	209	216	222	229	236	243
71	136	143	150	157	165	172	179	186	193	200	208	215	222	229	236	243	250
72	140	147	154	162	169	177	184	191	199	206	213	221	228	235	242	250	258
73	144	151	159	166	174	182	189	197	204	212	219	227	235	242	250	257	265
74	148	155	163	171	179	186	194	202	210	218	225	233	241	249	256	264	272
75	152	160	168	176	184	192	200	208	216	224	232	240	248	256	264	272	279
76	156	164	172	180	189	197	205	213	221	230	238	246	254	263	271	279	287

BMI

Height (inches)	36	37	38	39	40	41	42	43	44	45	46	47	48	49	50	51	52	53	54
							Body Weight (pounds)												
58	172	177	181	186	191	196	201	205	210	215	220	224	229	234	239	244	248	253	258
59	178	183	188	193	198	203	208	212	217	222	227	232	237	242	247	252	257	262	267
60	184	189	194	199	204	209	215	220	225	230	235	240	245	250	255	261	266	271	276
61	190	195	201	206	211	217	222	227	232	238	243	248	254	259	264	269	275	280	285
62	196	202	207	213	218	224	229	235	240	246	251	256	262	267	273	278	284	289	295
63	203	208	214	220	225	231	237	242	248	254	259	265	270	278	282	287	293	299	304
64	209	215	221	227	232	238	244	250	256	262	267	273	279	285	291	296	302	308	314
65	216	222	228	234	240	246	252	258	264	270	276	282	288	294	300	306	312	318	324
66	223	229	235	241	247	253	260	266	272	278	284	291	297	303	309	315	322	328	334
67	230	236	242	249	255	261	268	274	280	287	293	299	306	312	319	325	331	338	344
68	236	243	249	256	262	269	276	282	289	295	302	308	315	322	328	335	341	348	354
69	243	250	257	263	270	277	284	291	297	304	311	318	324	331	338	345	351	358	365
70	250	257	264	271	278	285	292	299	306	313	320	327	334	341	348	355	362	369	376
71	257	265	272	279	286	293	301	308	315	322	329	338	343	351	358	365	372	379	386
72	265	272	279	287	294	302	309	316	324	331	338	346	353	361	368	375	383	390	397
73	272	280	288	295	302	310	318	325	333	340	348	355	363	371	378	386	393	401	408
74	280	287	295	303	311	319	326	334	342	350	358	365	373	381	389	396	404	412	420
75	287	295	303	311	319	327	335	343	351	359	367	375	383	391	399	407	415	423	431
76	295	304	312	320	328	336	344	353	361	369	377	385	394	402	410	418	426	435	443

Appendix B
Three-Week Starter Plan

■　　■　　■　　■　　■

Week 1

Make Your Home Environment Work for You Instead of Against You

1. Clear your home of any problem foods (chips, cookies, ice cream, soda, and the like). If they are not available, you are less likely to eat them. You can still eat these foods, but it will be easier for you if they are not around the house. Stock your home with healthy and satisfying alternatives:

light string cheese	fat-free fudgsicles
skim milk	frozen fruit juice bars
low-fat cottage cheese	low-fat pudding
reduced-fat yogurt	sugar-free Jell-O
	bottled water
fruits	mineral water
vegetables	herbal tea
Mrs. Dash	
Garlic powder	cereals with fiber*
black pepper	whole-grain bagels*
Kosher salt	whole-grain waffles*
	low-fat granola bars*
light salad dressings	whole-grain bread*
olive oil	whole-grain crackers*
low-fat mayonnaise	whole-grain pasta*

brown rice*	soybeans (edamame)
light microwave popcorn	reduced-fat peanut butter
turkey slices	nutrition bars (Balance, Luna, Slim Fast) and drinks (Slim Fast)
tuna packed in water	Healthy Choice, Lean Cuisine, and Weight Watchers Smart
chicken breasts	Ones meals
bean soups	
beans and lentils	*Good source of fiber = 2.5–5 grams per serving; high-fiber =
Boca Burgers	more than 5 grams per serving.

2. Ask someone you trust for help. You need support. Be specific by asking that person to:
- be open-minded about sampling new and healthier foods
- become your walking or exercise buddy
- watch the kids so you can take time for yourself

Take Control of Your Eating

1. Don't go long periods (4–5 hours) without eating.
- Try to distribute your calories evenly throughout the day.
- Don't skip meals to save calories.
- Try eating breakfast if you don't already.

2. Eat more fruits and vegetables.
- Prepare fruits and vegetables so they are ready to eat.
- Buy precut or from the salad bar.
- Have a fruit bowl on the table.
- Make fruits and vegetables easy to grab and eat.
- Store fruits and vegetables in the front of the fridge where you see them first.
- Dip fruits and veggies in low-fat dressings and yogurt.

3. Carry a water bottle with you (hunger is often a sign of dehydration). Strive for eight 8-ounce glasses of water a day.
- Drink a glass when you wake up.
- Drink a glass with each meal.

- Drink a glass when you feel hungry.
- Never pass a water fountain without taking a drink.
- If you're getting bored with plain water, add a twist of lemon, lime, or orange.
- Try a no-calorie fruit-flavored water.
- Try mineral water.
- Use a colorful straw.

Take Control of Your Activity

1. Buy (and wear daily) a pedometer. This makes activity fun and helps you mark your progress. Be sure to buy one that counts steps, not miles. Most sporting goods stores carry them for under $30. Or you can order the Digi-Walker #AE120 from Accusplit in San Jose, California, 1-800-935-1996, ext. 204; www.accusplit.com.

Using your pedometer, record the number of steps taken per day for 2–3 days (preferably a weekday and a weekend day) and then calculate your average baseline. Once you've determined your baseline, you can begin to increase the number of steps taken by 500–750 (or 10 percent) over your baseline. You can accomplish this by:

- walking to a friend's house instead of driving
- taking your dog for longer walks
- doing your own housework or gardening

2. Get appropriate walking footwear (walking shoes or cross trainers). These are essential for injury-free walking.

3. If you have any medical limitations that may pose problems for increasing your activity, see your health professional and follow his or her advice.

Destress

1. Take a deep breath and slow down. Your goal is to focus on your day-to-day behaviors to help you reach your longer-term weight loss goal, not to add stress to your day.

2. Think about the stressors at home hindering you and talk to someone you trust about ways to overcome them.

3. Aim for improvement, not perfection.

Week 1 Checklist

_____ I cleared my home of problem foods and snacks.
_____ I stocked my home with healthy foods and snacks.
_____ I found a supportive person and asked for help.
_____ I'm not going long periods without eating.
_____ I'm eating more fruits and vegetables.
_____ I'm drinking more water.
_____ I'm wearing a pedometer.
_____ I have a good pair of walking shoes.
_____ My baseline steps per day range from _____ to _____ with an average of _____.
_____ I've accumulated an additional 500–750 steps (or 10%) over baseline daily.

How did you do with week 1? Grade yourself: _____
(A = did everything B = did 75% C = did 50% D = did 25% F = did nothing)
■ Which areas were hardest for you? _____ Eating _____ Activity _____ Coping
■ What would you like to improve? _____

Week 2

Make Your Daily Work Environment Work for You Instead of Against You

1. If you work outside your home:

■ Find someone supportive at work who can help you when the going gets tough, or bring daytime numbers of supportive people you can call.

■ Identify junk food temptations and distance yourself from them, if possible. Suggest to coworkers that candy or other treats be kept in the lunchroom (out of sight).

■ Toss a fresh fruit or vegetable into your briefcase every day (apple, pear, orange, banana, baby carrots, cherry tomatoes, jicama slices).

■ Bring your lunches from home, if possible, or order healthier ones. Find the nutritious choices on take-out menus: grilled chicken or lean turkey sandwich on whole-grain bread, bean or vegetable soup, veggie or turkey sub with mustard instead of mayo, Greek salad, bagel and hummus, baked potato. Call establishments to check if they have healthy alternatives (light mayo for tuna salad, low-fat cheese for sandwiches) not listed on the menu.

■ Take note of healthier options in vending machines: yogurt, popcorn, pretzels, broth-based soup, bottled water, fruit.

■ If you pass tempting vending machines on your way from your desk to the rest room, don't carry your wallet on these trips.

- Stock office drawer, briefcase, or fridge with an emergency supply of healthy foods: Nature Valley granola bars, high-fiber cereal in baggies, flavored rice cakes, nutrition bars, low-fat yogurt, light microwave popcorn.
- If you have a traveling job, plan ahead. Toss fresh fruit and nutrition bars in your briefcase; bring exercise clothes and gym shoes; try to stay in hotels that have a fitness center.

2. If you work at home:
- Keep fresh fruit and vegetables on the counter.
- Toss fresh fruit or veggies in your purse, backpack, or diaper bag every day.
- Assemble healthier lunches at home: lean turkey on whole-grain bread; bean or vegetable soup; bean, vegetable, or spinach salad; reduced-fat peanut butter and jelly on high-fiber bagel; tuna salad with reduced-fat mayo; Luna bar and reduced-fat yogurt mixed with fresh fruit.

Take Control of Your Eating

1. Downsize portions. Cut your main dish red meat, chicken, or fish protein portion by half, or the size of a deck of cards or a cassette (approximately 4 ounces), and eat more fruit, vegetable, and whole-grain side dishes so you don't go hungry. Instead of the supersize sandwich, choose the regular. In restaurants, split the entrée but order your own salad, take home half the entrée, or order lunch-size or appetizer portions for dinner with extra salad or vegetable.
2. Set aside time to eat and enjoy lunch each day to avoid hunger and balance your calories throughout the day when you're using them.

Take Control of Your Activity

1. Maximize daily physical activity (ADLs) in your work environment by building more steps into your normal workday. Increase your baseline steps by another 500–750 steps (or 10 percent) per day. Here's how:
- Park your car farther from your destination.
- Get off at an earlier bus stop.
- Take walking breaks instead of coffee breaks.
- Walk down the hall to speak with a coworker instead of E-mailing.

Record steps taken and find your new average for this phase.

2. Make a list of enjoyable ways to be more active.
■ Walk in a park or at the zoo.
■ Go window shopping.
■ Take a brisk walk with spouse after dinner.
■ Go bike riding with your child or a friend.

3. Make a list of 3–5 aerobic options you would find enjoyable:
■ exercise videos
■ aerobic dance class
■ stationary bike or biking
■ treadmill or power walking

Research how you will plan exercise into your daily schedule. Look for community centers, medical center fitness programs, the Y, parks, commercial fitness centers, and home-based options.

4. Schedule in your daily planner 20- to 30-minute walking sessions at least 2–4 times this week.

Destress

1. Think about the stressors in your daily work environment and talk to someone you trust about ways to overcome them. If stress at work is causing you to eat comfort foods at night, talk it out, ask for help, and practice deep-breathing relaxation exercises. If it's late-afternoon fatigue, plan ahead by having healthy alternatives nearby or taking a walk outside.
2. Practice using the STOP method for destressing: *S*low down, *T*ake a breath, *O*bserve, *P*lan. To break your automatic stress response, at the earliest signs of feeling stress, *slow down* the pace of whatever you're doing, *take* a breath to release tension and bring you back to the here and now, *observe* the situation as an outsider would, without emotions or attitude, and then *plan* a healthier way to react to the situation.
3. Practice deep-breathing exercises daily. Sit on the side of your bed, close

your eyes, and take slow, deep breaths in and out. Inhale slowly through your nose to the count of 4 and then exhale through your mouth to the count of 4. As you exhale, you may repeat a word to yourself, such as "health" or "peace," to help you focus. Practice for 2–4 minutes if you can.

Try this technique throughout the day (keeping your eyes open when you need to) whenever you feel stressed, anxious, or even just tired. Practice it while standing in a long line at the bank, while stopped in your car at a red light, or before responding to an angry customer on the phone. Or try this strategy when you feel compelled to eat a food that you know can put a drain on your health, or if you're not really hungry but the sight of food triggers your desire to eat.

Week 2 Checklist

_____ I've continued to work on week 1 behaviors and skills.
_____ I've asked for support at work.
_____ I'm more aware of junk food temptations in my daily work environment.
_____ I'm eating healthier lunches.
_____ I've stocked my daily work environment with healthy foods and snacks.
_____ When traveling, I plan ahead.
_____ I'm downsizing my food portions.
_____ My steps per day range from _____ to _____ with an average of _____.
_____ I've accumulated an additional 500–750 steps (or 10%) over baseline daily.
_____ I walked for 20–30 minutes at least 2–4 times this week.
_____ I made a list of aerobic exercise options.
_____ I've talked to a supportive person about ways to overcome stressors in my work environment.
_____ I practiced the STOP method for destressing.
_____ I practiced deep breathing.

How did you do with week 2? Grade yourself:_____
(A = did everything B = did 75% C = did 50% D = did 25% F = did nothing)
- Which areas were hardest for you? _____ Eating _____ Activity _____ Coping
- What would you like to improve? _____

Week 3

Make your Social Environment Work for You
Instead of Against You

1. When you go to social events, plan ahead.
- Bring your own healthy dish to the party.
- Bring your own snack to the movies.
- Split a small popcorn.
- Try not to go to a social event hungry.

2. Plan an active social event.
- Go to a museum.
- Make a golf date.
- Go to the zoo.
- Take a bike expedition.
- Go dancing.
- Help the local gardening club.

3. When dining out, plan ahead.
- Downsize, don't supersize.
- Read the whole menu before choosing.
- Split an entrée.
- Limit bread and chips before the meal.
- Use olive oil instead of butter.
- Choose broth or bean soup instead of cream soup.
- Use less cheese.
- Ask for an extra side vegetable.
- Order dressing and sauce on the side.
- Order baked, poached, or grilled instead of fried.

Take Control of Your Eating

1. Try some new and different foods or sample something you haven't eaten in a while.

- pizza with lots of vegetables (and easy on the cheese or none at all)
- grilled or roasted vegetables
- fresh berries
- whole wheat pasta
- whole-grain bread
- a new light salad dressing
- vinegars (balsamic, red wine, apple cider)
- new marinade for your chicken breast or fish
- new herbs and spices, dried or fresh
- different greens in salads: spinach, arugula, red leaf lettuce

2. Sample a soy product.

- veggie burgers
- soybeans (edamame)
- seasoned tofu
- soy milk
- soy nuts
- veggie ground round/soy crumbles
- soy cheese

3. Eat fish.

- tuna sandwich with low-fat mayo
- grilled fish Grecian style
- whole fish Asian style
- seafood kebab
- shrimp cocktail

Take Control of Your Activity

1. Boost your ADLs (activities of daily living).
- Increase the number of steps taken daily from last week.
- Pick and do one of the enjoyable activities you listed last week.

2. Shift your exercise into higher gear.
- Continue to schedule 20- to 30-minute walking sessions (or other aerobic exercise activity that you previously identified) 2–4 times this week.
- Pick up the pace, walking with a purpose, as if you have somewhere to go.
- Take walks with a coworker, friend, or family member.
- Decide on a place, time, and schedule for an exercise program.

Destress

1. Think about the social stressors hindering you and talk to someone you trust about ways to overcome them.
2. Practice using the STOP method for destressing and pay attention to when this method is most helpful.
3. Take mindful walks alone where you can focus on the sights, sounds, and smells of your surroundings.

4. Inventory your progress.
- What parts of this program have been hard and what parts have been easy?
- What has been the reaction of friends and family?
- Who has been supportive and who has been a saboteur?
- What life stressors have gotten in the way of your success?

5. Congratulate and reward yourself for completing this three-phase program.
- Treat yourself to a manicure.
- Do some power shopping.
- Take a long walk in the park.
- Go to a sporting event.
- See a movie with your family.
- Spend special time with a friend.

Week 3 Checklist

_____ I've continued to work on behaviors and skills from weeks 1 and 2.

_____ I planned ahead before social events.

_____ I planned ahead before dining out.

_____ I planned ahead before going to the movies.

_____ I made healthy requests at restaurants.

_____ I tried new foods.

_____ I sampled new meals.

_____ My steps taken per day now range from _____ to _____ with an average of _____.

_____ I walked for at least 20–30 minutes 2–4 times this week.

_____ I'm varying my walks.

_____ I'm enjoying walking more.

_____ I participated in an enjoyable activity.

_____ I talked to a supportive person about ways to overcome social stressors.

_____ The STOP method has helped me destress.

_____ I rewarded myself for completing this three-week program.

How did you do with week 3? Grade yourself:_____

(A = did everything B = did 75% C = did 50% D = did 25% F = did nothing)

- Which areas were hardest for you? _____ Eating _____ Activity _____ Coping

- What would you like to improve? _____

Weight Busters at a Glance

Unguided Grazer	Nighttime Nibbler	Convenient Consumer	Fruitless Feaster	Mindless Muncher	Hearty Portioner	Deprived Sneaker
Create a supporting structure	Redistribute calories	Downsize, don't supersize	Get fresh	From mindless to conscious	Pace your mind and body	Dismiss "cheating"
Just eat—and enjoy	Calorieproof your home	Divide and conquer	Color your plate	Quantify munching	Proportion your plate	Add satisfaction with fat and fiber
Connect hunger and fullness cues	Plan 1 nightly snack that satisfies	Find hidden calories	Appeal to your senses	Refresh with healthier alternatives	Be savvy about servings	Moderate your sweet tooth
Fill up on fiber and water	Reset your nighttime routine	Cooking, anyone?	Dare to go bare	Tame your triggers	Overcome portion traps	Socialize and enjoy

Hate-to-Move Struggler	Self-Conscious Hider	Inexperienced Novice	All-or-Nothing Doer	Set-Routine Repeater	Aches-and-Pains Sufferer	No-Time-to-Exercise Protester
Count all activity	Dress the part	Ease into stretching	Adopt a moderate mind-set	Change the pace	Set healthy boundaries	Add it naturally
Energize your body and mind	Break a sweat at home	Start smart	Get real	Surprise your body	Make it short and sweet	Make appointment with self
Find fun	Be inconspicuous	Mark progress	Understand triggers	Don't resist resistance	Go alternative	Multitask your exercise
Buddy up	Move and meditate	Build muscle	Enjoy building skills	Swim against the stream	Seek supervision	Ask for help

Weight Busters at a Glance

Emotional Stuffer	Low-Self-Esteem Sufferer	Persistent Procrastinator	Can't-Say-No Pleaser	Fast Pacer	Pessimistic Thinker	Unrealistic Achiever
■ Inventory food and mood	■ Be real about body image	■ Probe procrastination trait	■ Understand the disease to please	■ Notice life imbalances	■ Realize pessimism's perils	■ Trim goals
■ Acknowledge your feelings	■ Affirm yourself	■ Prompt yourself	■ Envision your yeses	■ Use mindfulness to self-correct	■ Turn I can't into I can	■ Focus on the process
■ Nurture emotions without food	■ Dismiss the judging committee	■ Make it manageable	■ Say no like a pro	■ Squeeze in support	■ Accentuate the positive	■ Redirect energies
■ Strengthen mind-body connection	■ Befriend your body	■ Enjoy small successes	■ Learn to delegate	■ Revitalize regularly	■ Treat yourself better	■ Accept limitations

Appendix C
Resources

Eating

All Recipes
www.allrecipes.com
recipes, complete with nutrition analyses, meal ideas, and cooking advice; site allows you to scale recipes

American Dietetic Association
www.eatright.org
information on nutrition, healthy lifestyle, and finding a registered dietitian near you

American Institute of Cancer Research
www.aicr.org
healthy recipes, free publications, and tips for good health

Center for Science in the Public Interest
www.cspinet.org
nonprofit consumer advocacy group that also publishes *Nutrition Action HealthLetter;* offers information on hot nutrition topics and rate-your-diet quizzes

Cooking Light
www.cookinglight.com
recipes, menu planning, and cooking tips

Dole Eat Five a Day for Better Health
www.dole5aday.com/Teachers/T_Index.html
reference center with consumer information on the phytochemical and nutrient contents of fruits and vegetables

International Tree Nut Council, Nutrition Committee
www.nuthealth.org
nut nutrition information, recipes, and cooking tips

Peapod
www.peapod.com
on-line grocery shopping and delivery service

The Phytopia Cookbook
www.phytopia.com
recipes and other information on phytochemicals in plant foods

Tufts University Nutrition Navigator
www.navigator.tufts.edu/index.html
rates nutrition Web sites for accuracy and content

Exercise

Accusplit
www.accusplit.com
1-800-935-1996, ext. 204
sells pedometers

American College of Sports Medicine
www.acsm.org
news releases and position statements on topics related to exercise science and sports
medicine

American Council on Exercise
www.acefitness.org
nonprofit organization that offers information on fitness, health clubs, and ACE
certification

Collage Video
www.collagevideo.com
1-800-433-6769
exercise videos to preview and order; free catalog

Fitness Wholesale
www.fwonline.com
1-888-FW-ORDER

exercise equipment (resistance bands or tubing, fitness balls, mats, steps, weights, heart rate monitors, books, exercise software music, videos); free catalog

International Association of Fitness Professionals
www.ideafit.com
fitness tips and information on fitness instructors

Junonia
www.junonia.com
1-800-586-6642
women's active wear size 14 and up

Coping

American Massage Therapy Association
www.amtamassage.org
massage therapist national locator service

Mind/Body Medical Institute
www.mbmi.org
1-617-632-9530
stress and wellness information, relaxation tapes

My Daily Yoga
www.mydailyyoga.com
pictures and descriptions of daily exercises

Psychology Today
www.psychologytoday.com
information on personal insights, relationships, health, and nutrition

Spa Finders
www.spafinders.com
information on day and stay spas; catalog

Volunteer Match
www.volunteermatch.org
volunteer opportunities across United States; includes virtual volunteering

Other Support and Professional Help

American Association of Lifestyle Counselors
www.aalc.org
1-817-545-3220
certified lifestyle counselors in your area

American Dietetic Association, Consumer Nutrition Hotline
1-800-366-1655
registered dietitians in your area

American Psychological Association
1-800-964-2000
mental health professionals near you

American Society of Bariatric Physicians
www.asbp.org
professional group of physicians with an interest in obesity

American Society of Bariatric Surgery
www.asbs.org
group established to advance the art and science of obesity surgery

Association for Morbid Obesity
www.obesityhelp.com
nonprofit organization providing peer support and resources for morbid obesity and
bariatric surgery

Heathetech
www.healthetech.com
information on their Palm or Windows software program for personalized weight
management

Northwestern Memorial Hospital Wellness Institute (Chicago)
www.nmh.org/classes/wellness_institute.html
information on their nutrition, weight management, fitness, stress management, and
smoking cessation programs and classes

Overeaters Anonymous
www.overeatersanonymous.org
information on its recovery program for overeating and on finding a group in your area

Take Off Pounds Sensibly
www.tops.org
information on its support group and on finding a chapter near you

General

American Heart Association
www.americanheart.org
heart-healthy lifestyle information on nutrition, shopping, dining out, and exercise

LEARN—The Lifestyle Company
www.learneducation.com
self-assessment weight loss and stress management tools and tips, book catalog

Mayo Clinic
www.mayoclinic.com
information on nutrition, vitamins, minerals, and herbal supplements

Medline Plus Health
www.nlm.nih.gov/medlineplus
information for consumers, a service of the National Library of Medicine/NIH

National Heart, Lung, and Blood Institute Obesity Education Initiative
www.nhlbi.nih.gov/about/oei/index.htm
selecting a weight loss program, menu planning, food label reading, and BMI calculation
and interpretation

National Weight Control Registry
www.uchsC.edu/nutrition/nwcr.htm
1-800-606-NWCR
ongoing datebase of successful weight loss maintainers

Shape Up America
www.shapeup.org
consumer-based site founded by past surgeon general C. Everett Koop, MD; information
on nutrition and fitness

U.S. Food and Drug Administration
www.fda.gov
1-888-463-6332
information on losing weight safely and food labeling

Weight Control Information Network
www.niddk.nih.gov/health/nutrit/win.htm
weight loss articles from the National Institutes of Health

Your Online Diet and Fitness Journal
www.fitday.com
helps you track different aspects of your diet, fitness, and weight, and even gives you
graphical reports

Selected Bibliography

Eating

American Dietetic Association, with Jean Pennington. *The Essential Guide to Nutrition and the Foods We Eat*. New York: Harper, 1999.

Chesman, Andrea. *The Roasted Vegetable*. Boston: The Harvard Common Press, 2002.

Food and Nutrition Board, Institute of Medicine. *Dietary Reference Intakes for Macronutrients*. Washington, D.C.: National Academy Press, 2002.

Frazao, Elizabeth, ed. *America's Eating Habits: Changes & Consequences*. Economic Research Service Report. Washington, DC: USDA, 1999.

Jacobson, Michael F., and Jayne Hurley. *Restaurant Confidential*. Workman Publishing Company, 2002.

Kennedy, Eileen T., et al. "Popular Diets: Correlation to Health, Nutrition, and Obesity." *Journal of the American Dietetic Association* 101 (2001): 411–19.

Madison, Deborah. *This Can't Be Tofu!* New York: Broadway Books, 2000.

McCrory, Megan A., et al. "Dietary Variety Within Food Groups: Association with Energy Intake and Body Fatness in Men and Women." *American Journal of Clinical Nutrition* 69 (1999): 440–47.

Miller, Gregory D., ed. "New Frontiers in Weight Management." *Journal of the American College of Nutrition* 21 (2002): 131S–155S.

Pennington, Jean. *A.T. Bowe's & Church's Food Values of Portions Commonly Used*. 17th ed. Philadelphia: Lippincott Raven, 1998.

Shapiro, Howard M. *Picture Perfect Weight Loss: The Visual Program for Permanent Weight Loss*. Emmaus, PA: Rodale, 2000.

Young, Lisa R., and Marion Nestle. "The Contribution of Expanding Portion Sizes to the US Obesity Epidemic." *American Journal of Public Health* 92 (2002): 246–249.

Exercise

Ainsworth, Barbara E., et al. "Compendium of Physical Activities: An Update of Activity Codes and MET Intensities." *Medicine and Science in Sports and Exercise* 32 (2000): S498–516.

American College of Sports Medicine. *ACSM's Guidelines for Exercise Testing and Prescription*. 6th ed. Philadelphia: Lippincott Williams & Wilkins, 2000.

Anderson, Bob. *Stretching*. 20th anniversary ed. Bolinas, CA: Shelter Publications, 2000.

Hurley, Ben F., and Stephen M. Roth. "Strength Training in the Elderly: Effects on Risk Factors for Age-Related Diseases." *Sports Medicine* 4 (October 30, 2000): 249–68.

Jakicic, John. M., et al. "Appropriate Intervention Strategies for Weight Loss and Prevention of Weight Regain for Adults." *Medicine and Science in Sports and Exercise* 33, 12 (2001): 2145–56.

Kraemer, William J., et al. "Progression Models in Resistance Training for Healthy Adults." *Medicine and Science in Sports and Exercise* 34, 2 (2002): 364–80.

Nelson, Miriam E., with Sarah Wernick. *Strong Women Stay Slim*. New York: Bantam, 1998.

Pate, Russell, et al. "Physical Activity and Public Health: A Recommendation from the Center for Disease Control and Prevention and the American College of Sports Medicine." *JAMA* 273, 5 (1995): 402–07.

Westcott, Wayne L., and Thomas R. Baechle. *Strength Training Past 50*. Champaign, IL: Human Kinetics, 1998.

Coping

Bertson, Herbert. *The Relaxation Response*. New York: Avon, 1975.

Borysenko, Joan. *Inner Peace for Busy People: 52 Simple Strategies for Transforming Your Life*. Carlsbad, CA: Hay House, 2001.

Braiker, Harriet B. *The Disease to Please: Curing the People-Pleasing Syndrome*. New York: McGraw-Hill, 2001.

Branden, Nathaniel. *The Six Pillars of Self-Esteem: The Definitive Work on Self-Esteem by the Leading Pioneer in the Field*. New York: Bantam, 1994.

Breathnach, Sarah Ban. *Simple Abundance: A Daybook of Comfort and Joy*. New York: Warner Books, 1995.

Breitman, Patti, and Connie Hatch. *How to Say No Without Feeling Guilty: And Say Yes to More Time, More Joy, and What Matters Most to You*. New York: Broadway Books, 2000.

Cash, Thomas F. *What Do You See When You Look in the Mirror? Helping Yourself to a Positive Body Image*. New York: Bantam, 1995.

Domar, Alice D. *Self Nurture: Learning to Care for Yourself as Effectively as You Care for Everyone Else*. New York: Viking, 2000.

Hafen, Brent Q., et al. *Mind/Body Health: The Effects of Attitudes, Emotions, and Relationships*. Needham Heights, MA: Allyn & Bacon, 1996.

Levey, Joel and Michelle. *Living in Balance: A Dynamic Approach for Creating Harmony & Wholeness in a Chaotic World*. Berkeley, CA: Conari Press, 1998.

Rodin, Judith. *Body Traps: Breaking the Binds that Keep You from Feeling Good*. New York: William Morrow, 1992.

Stedman, Nancy. "Stop Stressing!" *Redbook*, September 1999, p. 78.

Thayer, Robert E. *Calm Energy: How People Regulate Mood with Food and Exercise*. New York: Oxford University Press, 2001.

Van Cauter, Eve, et al. "Age-Related Changes in Slow Wave Sleep and REM Sleep and Relationship with Growth Hormone and Cortisol Levels in Healthy Men." *JAMA* 284 (2000): 861–68.

Villarosa, Linda. "New Fitness Guidelines Spur Debate on Fitness." *New York Times*, June 23, 1998.

General

Kushner, Robert F., Johanna J. Mytko, and Nancy Kushner. "Using a New Symptom Pattern Approach for Management of Obesity: Development of an Introductory Questionnaire." *American Journal of Clinical Nutrition* 75 (2002): 368S–69S.

Schneider, Karen S. "The Facts About Figures." *People Weekly* 45, 22 (1996).

Strote, Mary Ellen, and Courtney Rubin. "How America Is Making You Fat." *Shape*, March 2001, pp. 138–44.

Wing, Rena R., and James O. Hill. "Successful Weight Loss Maintenance." *Annual Review of Nutrition* 21 (2001): 323–41.

Index

Index